Outline of Cardiology

Outline of Cardiology

Second Edition

John Vann Jones PhD, FRCP

Consultant Cardiologist,
Royal Infirmary, Bristol

and

Roger Blackwood MA, FRCP

Consultant Physician, Wexham Park Hospital, Slough;
Honorary Consultant Physician and Cardiologist,
Hammersmith Hospital, London

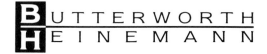
BUTTERWORTH
HEINEMANN

Butterworth-Heinemann Ltd
Linacre House, Jordan Hill, Oxford OX2 8DP

 PART OF REED INTERNATIONAL BOOKS

OXFORD   LONDON   BOSTON
MUNICH   NEW DELHI   SINGAPORE   SYDNEY
TOKYO   TORONTO   WELLINGTON

First published 1983
Second edition 1992
Reprinted 1992

British Library Cataloguing in Publication Data
A CIP catalogue record for this book is available from the British Library

Library of Congress Cataloguing in Publication Data
A CIP catalogue record for this book is available from the Library of Congress

ISBN 0 7506 1442 0

Composition by Genesis Typesetting, Laser Quay, Rochester, Kent
Printed and bound by Courier International Limited, East Kilbride

Contents

Preface

The purpose of the second edition of this book
remains the same as that of the first. We hope to
provide an up-to-date concise account of
cardiology. However, this edition has been aimed
specifically at medical students and junior hospital
doctors at the level of their first appointment. We
have extensively updated the treatment sections
because, of course, cardiology is a subject that has
changed markedly since the first edition of the
book. Some of the practical procedures have been
omitted this time, for example pacemaker insertion,
the practicalities of which have little relevance to
medical students.

As with the previous edition we have received a
lot of help, particularly from JVJ's secretary, Rita
Payne, who retyped the manuscript. Updated
echocardiograms have been provided by Dr Peter
Wilde. Once again we would like to thank our wives
for their forbearance and surprisingly their names
are still Anne and Libby.

J. V. J.
R. B.

Preface to the first edition

The purpose of this book is to provide a short concise account of modern cardiology with emphasis on common conditions and problems. It is intended for junior hospital doctors finding themselves in their first cardiology job or studying for higher medical qualifications. It should also be of interest to medical students, to nurses or other paramedical people involved with cardiology patients, and to physicians in more general units or in other specialties who want to know a little more about diseases of the heart and circulation. We have included rather detailed descriptions of certain cardiac procedures, e.g. pacemaker insertion, because this is the sort of thing that can be difficult to glean from elsewhere.

We started writing this book when we were colleagues at the John Radcliffe Hospital, Oxford, and rather surprisingly it survived our translation to other places. We received a large amount of help, of course, not least from our secretaries Karen Fryman, Alison Nicholls and Hilary Griffin and from Ken Browne who drew all our illustrations where these are not real records that have been reproduced directly. David Bennett from Wythenshawe Hospital, Manchester, another former colleague, provided many of the traces produced in Chapter 9 and, indeed, they were 'poached' from his own book 'Cardiac Arrhythmias'. Dr Frank Ross provided most of the echocardiograms in the book. Professor Peter Sleight financed much of the initial expense and we are very grateful for his support. Finally, we would like to thank our wives, Anne and Libby, for their forbearance and encouragement.

J. V. J.
R. B.

1

The heart and circulation

● **Anatomy and physiology**

Embryological development of the heart

The embryology of the heart is complex but basically starts with a single tube that has peristaltic action. At one end of the tube are gathered the veins (vitelline, cardinal and umbilical) and at the other end the arteries in the form of two dorsal aortae and six branchial arches. Remnants of these arches and aortae eventually go to form many parts of the vessels found in the adult or mature circulation, e.g. first – maxillary; second – stapedial; third – common carotid and proximal internal carotid; fourth – right subclavian and part of aorta; fifth – atrophies; sixth – pulmonary artery and ductus arteriosus (*Fig.* 1.1). The right dorsal aorta also becomes part of the right subclavian artery and the left dorsal aorta part of the aorta proper. It is soon obvious that there are four components to the heart tube, the sinus venosus, atria, ventricular inlet and ventricular outlet portions. Over the first 2 months the tube folds back on itself and rotates to the right. Septa appear and the great arteries form and migrate to their appropriate positions. The veins become incorporated partly into the atria and partly into the venae cavae. The basic human heart is formed in this way within the first 8 weeks of intrauterine life and it is hardly surprising that fairly frequently the development goes wrong.

In utero blood returns from the placenta to the right atrium where it either passes to the right ventricle and then to the pulmonary artery and then largely out across a patent ductus arteriosus, or it passes through the foramen ovale directly to the left atrium and hence to the systemic circulation. The pulmonary vascular resistance is high *in utero* encouraging blood to bypass the lungs and to go through the patent ductus (*Fig.* 1.2). At birth this resistance drops, the ductus and foramen ovale close and the adult pattern of circulation takes over (*Fig.* 1.3).

Cardiac anatomy

There are basically four cardiac chambers (*Fig.* 1.4). The superior and inferior venae cavae drain into the right atrium, a low pressure system with mean

1

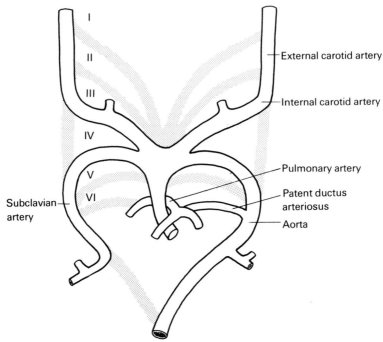

Fig. 1.1.   The branchial arches and the formation of the great vessels.

pressures ranging from negative values to about +6 mmHg. Higher pressures than this cause venous distension and engorgement of the liver. Blood from the right atrium crosses the tricuspid valve into the right ventricle where the pressure is normally less than 30 mmHg systolic and 0–6 mmHg diastolic. The right ventricle has traditionally been described as having an inlet portion and an outflow tract. The body of the ventricle itself is heavily trabeculated, much more so than the left ventricle which is relatively smooth by comparison. Blood is pumped by the right ventricle across the pulmonary valve into the pulmonary artery where the systolic pressure also should not exceed 30 mmHg. Pressures in the peripheral pulmonary arteries are lower than in the main pulmonary artery by a few mmHg.

After oxygenation in the lungs the blood returns to the left atrium via four pulmonary veins. The pressure here is a maximum mean of 12 mmHg and is therefore considerably higher than in the right atrium. This higher pressure early in life holds the foramen ovale functionally shut until it becomes permanently closed considerably later. This potential opening is of great help to the cardiologist because it usually means that in young infants a cardiac catheter can be inserted through the foramen ovale from the venous side of the heart.

Left atrial blood crosses the mitral valve into the left ventricle. Here pressures vary a lot with age but in adults the systolic pressure is at least

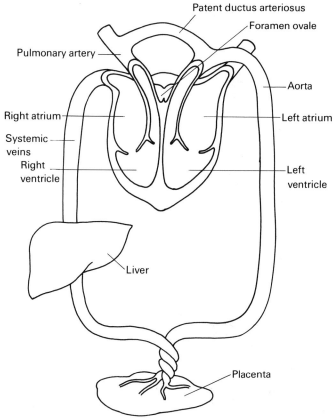

Fig. 1.2. The fetal circulation.

100 mmHg while at the end of diastole it should be less than 12 mmHg. An elevated end diastolic pressure is a useful indicator of left ventricular dysfunction. The left ventricle ejects its contents in systole over the aortic valve and into the aorta.

The heart's own blood supply comes from two major coronary arteries. The right coronary supplies the right atrium and right ventricle and a variable extent of the interventricular septum and inferior surface of the left ventricle. It also gives off a branch to the sino-atrial node. The left coronary soon divides into two major branches: the left anterior descending artery which runs down the anterior surface of the heart supplying the anterior left ventricle and apex, and the circumflex artery which runs in the atrioventricular groove at the back of the heart supplying the structures there. There are two points to be made about this anatomical arrangement. The first part of the left coronary, the left main, is a vitally important vessel. Atheroma in this part is extremely dangerous as occlusion of the artery at this point would have disastrous consequences for the

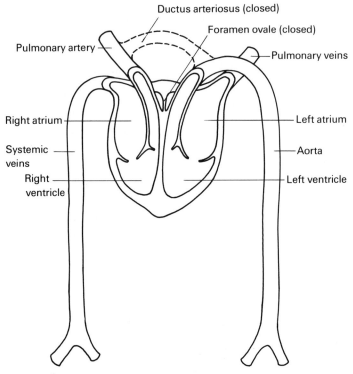

Ductus arteriosus (closed)

Foramen ovale (closed)

Pulmonary artery

Pulmonary veins

Right atrium

Left atrium

Systemic
veins

Aorta

Right
ventricle

Left ventricle

Fig. 1.3.   The mature circulation.

heart. In the atrioventricular groove the left circumflex artery lies beside the large coronary sinus and there is danger of damaging this vein at surgery. In addition the circumflex, lying as it does at the back of the heart, is in any event relatively inaccessible to the surgeon when compared with the other vessels (*Fig.* 1.5).

The heart has its own system of veins running in parallel with the main arteries. They finally drain into the coronary sinus which itself drains directly into the right atrium. There is also a lymphatic system, the anatomy and function of which is little understood but it eventually drains into the thoracic duct.

The heart has four valves (*Fig.* 1.4). Those between the atria and the ventricles are the tricuspid and mitral valves. These are referred to as the atrioventricular (AV) valves and the first heart sound results from their closure at the start of systole. The second heart sound marks the end of systole and is due to the aortic and pulmonary valves closing. The aortic valve usually closes first as the high pressure aorta slams it closed. The pulmonary valve tends more to drift shut. Thus, the second heart sound is split with an aortic and pulmonary component audible. On inspiration this splitting is marked as more blood returns to the right side of the heart and delays pulmonary valve closure. Splitting of the

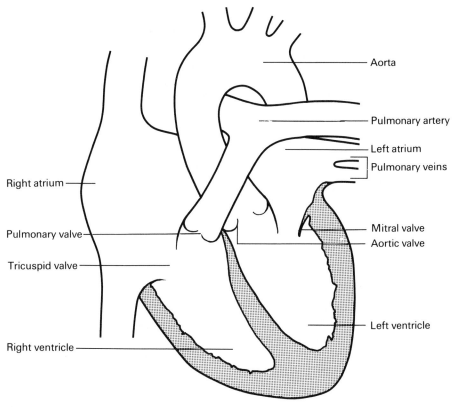

Fig. 1.4.   The anatomy of the normal heart.

second heart sound is particularly well heard in children and its absence or lack of variation should make you look more closely for heart disease.

Cardiac physiology

The heart's basic function is to pump, but there are four such pumps which must work in proper sequence. In order to do this the pump has an internal wiring system that allows a proper sequence of filling, pumping and emptying. In addition there are escape mechanisms to allow for failure of any part of the internal wiring system and there are external nerves which can alter the performance of the pump depending on the needs of the body as a whole. As a final refinement there are receptors in the heart that can modify its performance and alter and respond to its work load.

The heart as a series of pumps

The heart is best considered as two separate atrial pumps emptying into two ventricular pumps. Venous blood returns to the heart largely due to the

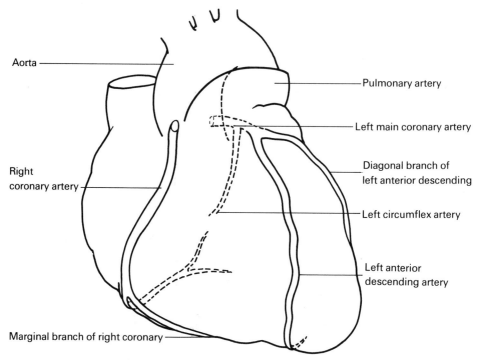

Aorta

Pulmonary artery

Left main coronary artery

Right
coronary artery

Diagonal branch of
left anterior descending

Left circumflex artery

Left anterior
descending artery

Marginal branch of right coronary

Fig. 1.5.   The coronary arteries.

negative intrathoracic pressure and to the skeletal muscle pumps compressing systemic veins. The atria fill passively but when they contract they tend to nip off the venae cavae so that blood, in the main, passes through the AV valves into the ventricles. The timing of atrial contraction is such that it occurs late in diastole and therefore really just primes the ventricle with a last top up. In other words 80–90 per cent of venous return comes back to the atria, runs into the ventricles when the AV valves open and then finally the atria contract to pass another 10–20 per cent of the venous return into the appropriate ventricle. Therefore in health atrial systole contributes up to 20 per cent of cardiac output. Where the ventricle is diseased or heart valves are damaged atrial systole can be much more important. For instance it has been estimated that in patients surviving a myocardial infarction atrial systole may contribute to as much as 50 per cent of the cardiac output.

With atrial systole there is some regurgitation into the systemic veins. This is seen as the 'a' wave in the jugular venous pulse; 'v' waves are also seen in time with ventricular systole but the exact mechanism of how they occur is under debate.

When the ventricles start to contract they close the AV valves as the intraventricular pressure rises. The ventricles effectively clamp round their

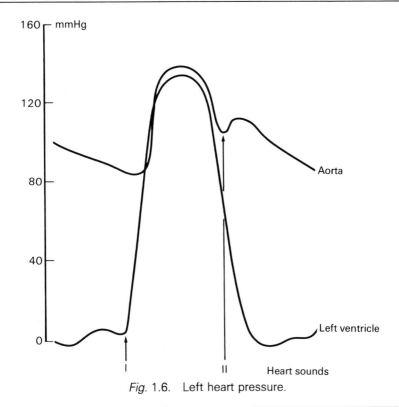

Fig. 1.6.   Left heart pressure.

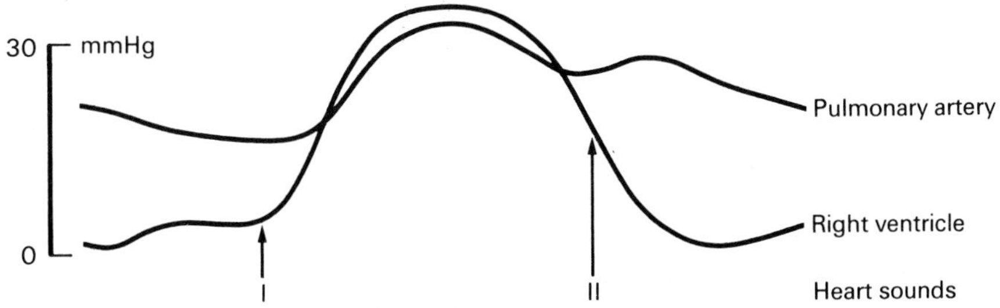

Fig. 1.7.   Right heart pressures.

contents (the period of isovolumic contraction) and the pressure rises rapidly until it exceeds the aortic or pulmonary artery pressure. The contents are then ejected (isometric contraction) and aortic and pulmonary pressures soon are greater than ventricular, the appropriate valves close and the ventricles relax. The cycle is then repeated (*Figs.* 1.6 and 1.7).

When blood is ejected into the aorta it distends the aorta which then recoils to force blood out into the peripheral arteries. As the aortic valve closes a notch, the dicrotic notch, appears on the pressure trace.

The Frank–Starling mechanism

Two physiologists (Otto Frank and Ernest Starling) made many of the basic observations on intrinsic control mechanisms of the heart nearly 100 years ago. It is now known that even the denervated heart exerts a great deal of control over its own performance. There are three important physiological points:

1.   If venous return increases, cardiac output increases.
2.   If left atrial pressure increases, cardiac output increases.
3.   When blood pressure rises, stroke volumes and cardiac output decrease. This fall in cardiac output with increased peripheral resistance can be compensated for by an increased filling pressure.

It is not difficult to see, therefore, why left atrial pressure has to be higher than right atrial pressure because the systemic vascular resistance (and pressure) is higher than the pulmonary vascular resistance (and pressure). Thus both sides of the heart are operating this basic control mechanism and although pressures are different, in this way cardiac output remains the same and in balance. As an example of this imagine the aorta being clamped. Stroke volume of the left ventricle falls because of the increased pressure. The lungs would rapidly fill with blood if the right ventricle kept up its output. The reduced venous return, however, reduces right atrial filling pressure and right ventricular output within a beat or two so that the two pumps are once more back in balance.

Starling's law of the heart states that as left ventricular end diastolic pressure increases (left atrial pressure) then cardiac output will increase in line

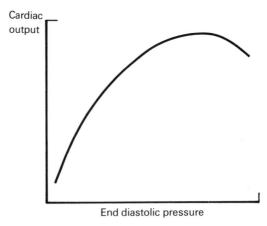

Fig. 1.8.   The Frank–Starling curve in a normal heart.

with this provided the peripheral resistance is unchanged (*Fig.* 1.8). However, there is a limit to how far this can go and eventually the end diastolic pressure is so great and the filling so excessive the heart cannot cope. At this stage we talk of the descending limb of the Starling curve. Such a situation is seen in patients with clinical left ventricular failure.

When heart rate increases stroke volume is reduced and cardiac output stays constant, provided there is no change in peripheral resistance (*Fig.* 1.9). As the heart speeds up diastole is shortened and diastolic filling time reduced. Eventually, however, diastole is so short that cardiac filling is ineffective and cardiac output will fall. Such a situation is sometimes seen in patients with fast cardiac arrhythmias and explains why they feel faint or dizzy or may even lose consciousness.

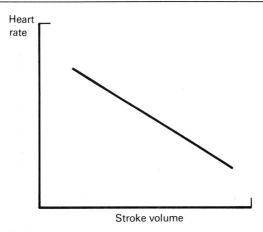

Fig. 1.9.   Relationship between heart rate and stroke volume at constant blood pressure.

Although the heart has a great range of control over its own performance as an inherent property of the muscle itself, it is also influenced by extrinsic factors such as circulating catecholamines, parasympathetic and sympathetic nerves.

Extrinsic control mechanisms

The heart has an extrinsic innervation, mostly to the regions of the sino-atrial and atrioventricular nodes. This is both sympathetic and parasympathetic and there is a complex interplay between these two influences when the heart rate changes. The parasympathetic (vagal) discharge slows the heart (sometimes to the level of ventricular standstill or various degrees of heart block) while sympathetic discharge increases heart rate. In the normal resting situation the vagal or parasympathetic influence is dominant.

Circulating catecholamines increase myocardial contractility and cause a tachycardia. In particular the contractility of atrial muscle is improved so that there is increased ventricular filling and hence cardiac output is increased over and above that resulting from the increased heart rate.

In the denervated heart the cardiac muscle fibres have to be stretched to increase their contractility (up to a certain limit as shown by the Starling curve). Catecholamines improve myocardial contractility without increased stretch of muscle fibres so that there is an effective shift of the Starling curve to the left. Of course sympathetic activity and catecholamines also affect the peripheral vasculature and the net result of sympathetic stimulation on cardiac performance depends upon the interplay of these various factors.

Cardiac receptors

There are receptors throughout the myocardium that greatly influence, reflexly, its performance. The atrial receptors, whose impulses are then carried in myelinated nerve fibres, have been classified as type A and type B. Type A discharge in atrial systole and seem to respond to atrial wall tension while type B respond to venous distension of the atria. Activation of atrial receptors may cause tachycardia and an increase in urinary output possibly by inhibition of antidiuretic hormone (ADH) secretion. Left atrial stretch may also release atrial natriuretic peptide (ANP), a substance that promotes sodium loss from the kidney. There are also atrial receptors with unmyelinated afferent fibres, discharging in response to atrial distension.

Ventricular receptors with both myelinated and unmyelinated afferent fibres have been described. The myelinated fibres are fewer and located at the apex. They may serve to prevent gross over-distension of the heart. Unmyelinated receptors are more widespread in the left ventricle and seem to respond to the level of end diastolic pressure. Both these receptors, when activated, result in negative inotropism (reduction in contractility) and negative chronotropism (reduction in heart rate). There are many other powerful reflex influences on the heart from receptors elsewhere, e.g. the peripheral arterial baroreceptors, the chemoreceptors and pulmonary or lung receptors. All of these can alter sympathetic or parasympathetic discharge to the heart

Electrical conduction in the myocardium (*Fig.* 1.10)

The pacemaker of the heart lies in the sino-atrial (SA) node at the junction of the superior vena cava and right atrium. Electrical impulses then pass through the atrial muscle, but not by any established pathway, to the atrioventricular (AV) node. Here there is an inbuilt delay mechanism and then the impulse passes to the bundle of His and then out to the right and left bundle branches. There is no anatomical justification for dividing the left bundle into anterior and posterior divisions as has been done by cardiologists although from the functional point of view this is a useful division. The left bundle is extensive and blocks may occur in it at various parts and it is useful to have nomenclature to describe this.

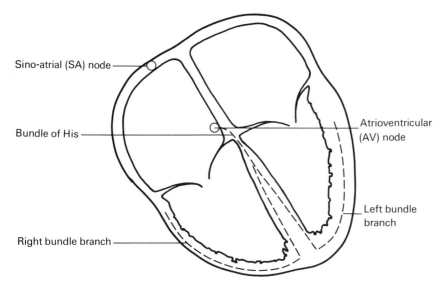

Fig. 1.10.   Intracardiac conduction pathways.

The passage of electricity through the atria corresponds to the P wave of the ECG. Delay in the AV node gives the isoelectric period between P wave and QRS. The QRS itself results from depolarization of all the ventricular muscle fibres while the T wave is ventricular muscle being repolarized. Repolarization of atrial muscle is lost in the QRS complex while a U wave is seen after the T wave in some individuals. Its cause is not known.

Electrical events at cellular level

When a microelectrode is inserted into a cardiac muscle cell the action potential recorded is altogether different from that seen with skeletal muscle. *Fig.* 1.11 shows a typical cardiac muscle action potential although this differs in different parts of the heart. For instance it is usually of less duration in atrial and conducting tissue fibres. This example would be more typical of a ventricular muscle cell.

There are two important things to note about this action potential. First of all it has a plateau which makes the action potential of long duration (300 ms+). Thus there is a limit to how fast the cell can beat. Unlike with skeletal muscle tetany cannot be induced in cardiac muscle by repeated stimuli; each contraction is separate. Another stimulus can evoke an action potential at certain points in this pattern (relative refractory period). This is noteworthy because at this point the myocardial cell is unstable and arrhythmias may result. Many anti-dysrhythmic drugs have their mode of action on different parts of the action potential. The second point to note is that between action potentials there is a steady rate of electrical leakage (depolarization) so that at a certain point

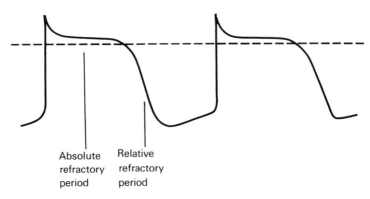

Absolute   Relative
refractory refractory
period   period

Fig. 1.11.   Action potential in a cardiac muscle cell.

(*Fig.* 1.11) another action potential becomes inevitable. This leakage can be affected by autonomic nerves, catecholamines and drugs as well as by electrolyte balance. The rate of leakage varies but is fastest in tissues of the SA node so that it is the effective heart pacemaker. It does mean that other muscle fibres can take over as pacemakers if the SA node is damaged.

The exact ionic changes that accompany the action potential are not known for certain but initially there seems to be a rapid influx of sodium into the cell followed by a slow influx of calcium. Potassium is lost fairly rapidly to begin with and then almost halfway through the action potential it moves back into the cell. During the slow decay period between action potentials potassium is lost from the cells and sodium enters. These events are of importance to the pharmacology of new drugs and already a large group (the calcium antagonists) have been developed as a result of this knowledge. Calcium does, of course, have profound effects on myocardial contractility with the result that different members of the calcium antagonist group have relatively greater or lesser effects on conduction or contractility in the heart.

Peripheral blood vessels

The heart has two sources of work. It has to take blood that is delivered to it and pass it onto either the body or the lungs. This is called the *preload* of the heart and is largely determined by venous return and the capacitance of the veins. If the veins are dilated venous return falls, preload is reduced and cardiac work is reduced. When the heart ejects blood the resistance to this is called the *afterload* and is a function of the arterial vessels, especially the small resistance vessels. Thus, not only do arteries and veins deliver and collect blood from the various tissues and organs but they can themselves greatly influence cardiac performance. When afterload is reduced stroke volume and cardiac output can increase markedly. The situation with preload is more complex depending on whether the heart is healthy or not. Once again knowledge of this pathophysiology has led to therapeutic developments and vasodilators in the treatment of heart failure either by preload or afterload reduction or both are established drugs.

The blood vessels are under nervous control, much of it reflex in origin. There are alpha-adrenergic receptors which result in vasoconstriction and beta-adrenergic receptors which result in vasodilatation. Nervous influences are greater on the arterial side but the veins are assuming more importance as we understand more about their physiology. The veins, for instance, contain two-thirds of the circulating blood volume at any one time. This compares with approximately one-eighth in the arteries and one-tenth in the lungs. It is evident therefore that small changes in venous capacity can have profound changes on circulatory function overall.

Ultrastructure of the heart

The heart resembles skeletal muscle in that it is striated, i.e. at microscopy it shows alternate light and dark bands. This is due to the arrangement of actin and myosin filaments within the muscle cells. These filaments slide over one another when the cell is depolarized and cause contraction – the sliding filament theory. This process requires energy and is heavily dependent upon calcium ions.

Cardiac muscle cells are connected one to another by structures called intercalated discs. These discs allow the easy passage of action potentials from one cell to the next so that their electricity can pass throughout the myocardium with extreme rapidity.

Myocardial cells form a syncytium round the ventricular cavities. The cells are arranged in a manner rather resembling wool wound up into a ball. This makes for efficient and relatively uniform contraction down onto the ventricular cavity and its contents with each systole.

2

Symptoms of heart disease

Careful history taking is very important in cardiology. For example the diagnosis of angina pectoris is made on the history alone and not on examination or tests. The catch phrase is 'listen to the patient, he is telling you the diagnosis'.

Cardiovascular disease may be very severe without symptoms. A myocardial infarction may be totally silent and aortic stenosis may be very tight indeed and the patient asymptomatic. Generally speaking, however, the severity of symptoms is proportional to the degree of disease. This can be a useful guide in the timing of cardiac surgery. For instance, when a patient with mitral stenosis can no longer climb a flight of stairs without stopping, valve surgery is almost certainly indicated.

There are numerous cardiac symptoms but pain, breathlessness in some form, palpitations, syncope and fatigue are probably the commonest.

● Dyspnoea

Shortness of breath (dyspnoea) is very subjective and therefore individual variation is great. What may be incapacitating to one patient may be largely ignored by another. Breathlessness is described by the patient either as a feeling of suffocation and the need to take another breath or having to breathe more deeply to feel comfortable. The physiology is complex but in simple terms the sensation of breathlessness is caused by increased stiffness of the lungs. In heart disease this means an increased volume of blood in the lungs (pulmonary congestion).

In practice it is important to determine the effort tolerance of a patient. The grading system of the New York Heart Association is commonly used.

Grade 1. Asymptomatic.
Grade 2. Symptoms obvious on moderate exercise.
Grade 3. Symptoms obvious on mild exercise.
Grade 4. Symptoms at rest.

Such a grading is useful and need not only apply to dyspnoea, but its disadvantage is that it is very imprecise. Subdivision of this grading has been attempted but it is still probably better to record what the patient actually says, i.e. breathless at 100 m, stops after three stairs, etc.

It must be remembered that a sedentary life, obesity and increasing age may limit exercise tolerance and causes other than cardiac ones may be present, e.g. anaemia, respiratory disease, metabolic changes.

Dyspnoea is probably the commonest cardiac symptom and in itself does not suggest a specific lesion. Dyspnoea may occur very late in a disease, e.g. aortic stenosis, when its presence is prognostically serious, but usually its severity gradually increases with that of the lesion.

Sudden dyspnoea suggests pulmonary embolism, acute pulmonary oedema, pneumothorax or an acute chest infection. Variable dyspnoea is usually psychogenic in origin and is often accompanied by an inability to get enough air into the lungs and periodic deep sighing. It can be helpful to get the patient to talk. In true dyspnoea they remain breathless and find talking difficult while in dyspnoea of psychogenic origin the breathlessness often improves markedly only to return afterwards. Nervously induced dyspnoea like this is often called hyperventilation.

● **Orthopnoea**

Orthopnoea is the sense of breathlessness when lying flat. It usually develops after dyspnoea is present and suggests a more severe form of cardiac lesion. When a patient lies down as much as 500 ml more blood are in the lungs compared with when standing. The lungs thus become stiffer. The patient does not lie flat in bed but props himself up with numerous pillows or decides to sleep in a chair. Often when he does fall asleep propped up he wakes up feeling uncomfortable after sliding down the bed (*Fig.* 2.1)

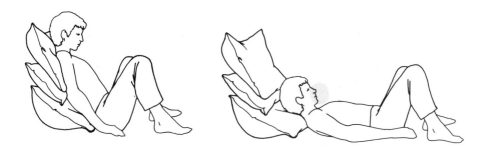

Fig. 2.1.   Orthopnoea.

● **Paroxysmal nocturnal dyspnoea**

In a typical episode, paroxysmal nocturnal dyspnoea occurs in the early hours of the morning when the patient awakes from his sleep gasping for breath with a feeling of suffocation. He sits upright and may climb out of bed and open a window to get cool air. The breathlessness may last from a few minutes to half an hour and is very distressing. The patient may feel he is going to die. Coughing and wheezing may be apparent and the cause of paroxysmal nocturnal dyspnoea is pulmonary oedema. It represents a serious symptom requiring urgent treatment (*Fig.* 2.2).

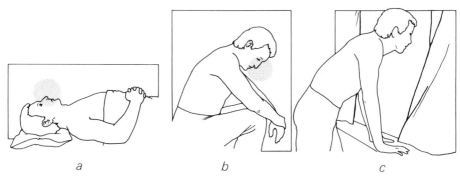

a   *b*   *c*

Fig. 2.2. (a)Paroxysmal nocturnal dyspnoea (PND). The patient wakens breathless and sits up (b) and then, very often, seeks fresh air, classically by opening a window (c).

● **Chest pain**

Chest pain is a most frightening symptom. The patient assumes he has serious cardiac disease if he develops any sort of chest pain and it is the physician's main objective to exclude this cause of pain if possible.

Cardiac pain may be in the form of angina pectoris or accompanying a myocardial infarct or unstable angina. The pain of angina pectoris is substernal, tight chest pain which sometimes radiates to the neck, jaw and one or both arms, usually the left arm. It is relieved by rest and may be associated with breathlessness, sweating and nausea. Angina pectoris will be dealt with in greater detail in chapter 8.

The pain of myocardial infarction or unstable angina is similar but very severe and crushing (*Fig.* 2.3).

While this description seems fairly clear it is far from easy on many occasions to decide whether chest pain is cardiac in origin or not. Cardiac pain is cosmopolitan in its presentation and detailed investigations may be necessary to decide if a patient really does have heart disease.

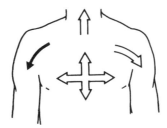

Fig. 2.3.   'Typical' distribution of pain in ischaemic heart disease.

Sublingual glyceryl trinitrate (GTN) relieves the pain of angina pectoris within 2–3 minutes but it cannot be used as a 'test' to see if the patient has angina. GTN will relax smooth muscle elsewhere, e.g. oesophageal spasm.

The patient will describe cardiac pain with a swoop of his hand across his chest. If he points to the pain with a finger it is unlikely to be cardiac pain which is rarely so localized.

The cause of cardiac pain is ischaemia of the myocardium. The commonest cause of this is coronary atheroma *per se* or occasionally associated coronary artery spasm. However, other causes must be considered: aortic stenosis, severe pulmonary stenosis, occasionally mitral valve disease and, now very rarely, syphilis. Pericardial pain (caused by pericarditis) is central, often very severe, but differs from angina by being affected by respiration. Many patients with pericarditis characteristically obtain relief from their pain by sitting forwards.

Quite different from these pains is the common left-sided inframammary pain, often innocent. Patients worried about their hearts may develop this pain which is stabbing in nature and not related to exercise. It was first described by Da Costa in the American Civil War in soldiers who for one reason or another considered they had heart disease. It was prominent in both World Wars but still is very common in peace-time. It has also been described as 'effort syndrome' or 'cardiac neurosis'. Similar pains however do occur with the billowing mitral leaflet syndrome when they may not always be innocent.

Other causes of chest pain must be distinguished from cardiac pain, e.g. pleural, oesophageal, gastric, duodenal, gall bladder, mediastinal and spinal as well as pain from chest wall ligaments and muscles (*Fig.* 2.4).

● **Palpitations**

Palpitation is an awareness of the beating of the heart and is not always pathological. After exercise or excitement thumping in the region of the heart is often felt.

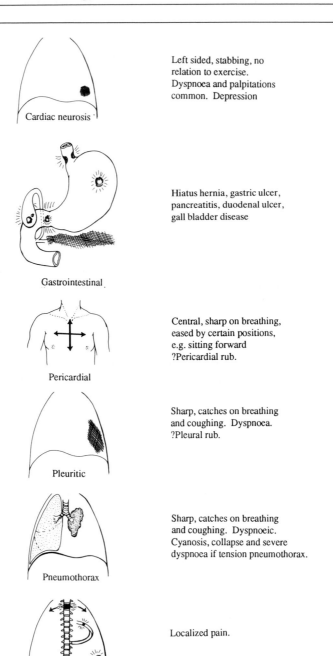

Left sided, stabbing, no
relation to exercise.
Dyspnoea and palpitations
common. Depression

Cardiac neurosis

Hiatus hernia, gastric ulcer,
pancreatitis, duodenal ulcer,
gall bladder disease

Gastrointestinal

Central, sharp on breathing,
eased by certain positions,
e.g. sitting forward
?Pericardial rub.

Pericardial

Sharp, catches on breathing
and coughing. Dyspnoea.
?Pleural rub.

Pleuritic

Sharp, catches on breathing
and coughing. Dyspnoeic.
Cyanosis, collapse and severe
dyspnoea if tension pneumothorax.

Pneumothorax

Localized pain.

Musculoskeletal

Fig. 2.4.   Common causes of chest pain not due to myocardial ischaemia.
(Reproduced with permission of Churchill Livingstone.)

The commonest palpitation is a heavy regular beating of the heart usually at a rate of about 100/min. This is produced by an excess of catecholamines and is related to stress or excitement. In itself it is quite innocent.

Other palpitations are divided into three groups.

'Missed' beats

This palpitation is caused by an ectopic (or premature) beat. The patient complains that his heart suddenly stopped and wondered if it was going to start again and that he felt a sudden heavy thump in the heart. This thump is not the ectopic beat, but the post-ectopic beat. A long diastolic period preceding the post-ectopic beat gives it a large stroke volume which is sensed quite differently from the normal beat. Such ectopics are common, often multiple, and can be normal or pathological.

Atrial ectopics are usually normal, occurring at times of stress or anxiety and sometimes associated with excessive coffee drinking or cigarette smoking. They may occur after a bout of heavy drinking, and are usually perceived at rest and disappear on exercise. Occasionally atrial ectopics are pathological and may go on to a supraventricular arrhythmia. Such a situation could occur with mitral stenosis. In the absence of anything else to suggest heart trouble (including the ECG) atrial ectopics can be assumed to be innocent and the patient strongly reassured.

Ventricular ectopics are slightly more likely to be pathological but are about as common as one's age, i.e. 50 per cent of 50-year-olds will have ventricular ectopics on a 24-hour ECG tape recording, 70 per cent of 70-year-olds and so on. Examination and the ECG may sometimes reveal evidence of ischaemic heart disease or other cardiac pathology. Treatment and causes of ventricular ectopics will be dealt with in chapter 9.

Fast heart rates

A very common complaint of a patient with palpitation is 'fluttering of the heart'. Supraventricular or ventricular tachycardias will produce sudden fluttering sensations in the chest often associated with a light-headed feeling, pallor, sweating and occasionally chest pain. Once it is established that a tachycardia is the palpitation two questions should be asked:

1. 'Did the fluttering come on gradually or suddenly?' Supraventricular tachycardias typically start suddenly while tachycardias due to fear or fright start more gradually. Similarly supraventricular tachycardias usually stop suddenly although this may be less obvious than the abrupt start.
2. 'Was the rhythm regular or irregular?' By tapping out with your pen on the table a regular rapid rhythm or an irregular rapid rhythm the patient may help you decide if the arrhythmia was regular (e.g. supraventricular tachycardia (SVT) or irregular (e.g. atrial fibrillation). In practice the patients are often too frightened to have noticed the rhythm but it is occasionally helpful.

Slow heart rates

This is a much rarer arrhythmia but the patient may complain of a slow heavy thumping in the chest. This would make one suspicious of complete heart block, but this abnormality is rarely perceived by the patient.

Despite a careful history, a routine 12-lead ECG is essential in all cases of palpitation and a 24-hour ECG tape or event marker may well be necessary.

● **Fatigue**

Fatigue is common in any illness. In heart disease it is an accompaniment to many other symptoms and is normally manifest as a 'physical tiredness'. For example, a child with cyanotic congenital heart disease will not play very much with other children because he cannot keep up with them. An adult with severe mitral stenosis may sleep every afternoon as well as 8–10 hours every night. The patient may complain of heaviness in the limbs on exertion, weakness or lack of vigour, or general tiredness and exhaustion. Fatigue is a highly subjective phenomenon made worse by anxiety, and is thus a very difficult symptom to assess. Nonetheless, those who have had a myocardial infarction often say that they noticed excessive fatigue in the preceding few months.

In cardiac failure, fatigue may be produced by a reduction in blood flow to skeletal muscle associated with histological and histochemical changes in the muscle cells. This may be an adaptive reaction of the body preventing the patient with failure from doing too much exercise.

● **Lightheadedness**

It is important to distinguish between lightheadedness and dizziness. Lightheadedness is a feeling of impending faintness and is often cardiac in origin although may be caused by extracardiac conditions, e.g. vertebrobasilar insufficiency. Dizziness refers to vertigo when the patient perceives the world spinning round, e.g. Ménière's disease. Lightheadedness of cardiac origin is due to a fall in cardiac output and syncope (loss of consciousness) may ultimately occur. Any lightheadedness followed by a focal neurological lesion, e.g. dysphasia, is rarely, if ever, due to a cardiac cause.

● **Syncope**

The sudden cessation of consciousness due to any cause is called syncope. It may be permanent or, more hopefully, transient, and a cardiac cause is only one such possibility. The cardiac causes are:

1.   Cardiac standstill – vagal inhibition.
2.   Ventricular asystole – a Stokes–Adams attack.
3.   Ventricular fibrillation.
4.   Atrial tachycardias.
5.   Aortic stenosis.
6.   Massive pulmonary embolism.
7.   Cardiac compression from haemopericardium.
8.   Low output state, e.g. shock, the cyanotic spells of Fallot's tetralogy.
9.   Prosthetic valve thrombosis.

Most of these conditions will lead to the patient being admitted to hospital as an emergency but two types of syncope may present in outpatients.

A Stokes–Adams attack is one where the patient falls abruptly to the ground without any warning, often injuring himself. Consciousness is frequently regained 2–3 minutes later with the patient feeling completely well apart from any injury he may have sustained as a result of falling down. The attacks occur when the patient goes into complete heart block during which periods of asystole suddenly present. It may also occur in the sick sinus syndrome. An artificial pacemaker will prevent these attacks.

Syncope associated with aortic stenosis is serious. The attack may be similar to a Stokes–Adams attack but there is usually some preceding lightheadedness. Once syncope has occurred in aortic stenosis death is likely within 2 years, even if there are no other symptoms, unless a valve replacement is performed.

All these forms of syncope occur independent of body position. Syncope occurring when the patient stands from the sitting or lying position is called postural hypotension. Its commonest cause is usually drugs, e.g. hypotensive agents. Micturition syncope or cough syncope is vagal in origin and may be accentuated by postural hypotension, e.g. the patient who gets out of bed at night and blacks out in the toilet.

Hysterical fainting usually occurs with no change in the pulse, blood pressure or colour of the patient or evidence of preceding symptoms. It may be associated with hyperventilation when the patient may complain of paraesthesiae of the hands and face.

● **Oedema**

As congestive heart failure develops fluid accumulates outside the tissues and causes swelling. Such fluid is under the influence of gravity and in the mobile patient ankle swelling develops. Because the swelling is fluid, pressure from a finger will cause it to 'pit' and the sign is known as pitting oedema. In the bedfast patient the effect of gravity is also to accumulate fluid over the sacrum.

In extreme cases oedema may spread right up the thighs and fluid may accumulate in the abdomen (ascites). Oedema is a sign of congestive cardiac failure but is also found in renal and hepatic failure, hypoproteinaemic states and where local blockage prevents adequate drainage, e.g. deep venous thrombosis or lymph drainage abnormalities. Dependent or stasis oedema may occur in the elderly patient and is of no pathological significance.

● **Cough**

Pulmonary oedema will manifest as a dry, non-productive cough, often particularly irritating during the night. In extreme cases the patient will cough up a pink frothy sputum and may be extremely breathless.

Coughing up blood (haemoptysis) occurs in advanced heart disease. As the pulmonary venous and left atrial pressures rise with severe heart disease, particularly congenital heart disease and mitral stenosis, the rupturing of a blood vessel will give distressing haemoptysis. With the advent of cardiac surgery this is a rare symptom and other causes (e.g. pulmonary embolus) are far more common.

A dry irritating cough is not infrequently observed with angiotensin converting enzyme inhibiting drugs, e.g. captopril, which are, of course, themselves often used to treat patients with chronic pulmonary oedema.

3

Examination of the cardiovascular system

● **Examination**

In examining any system in the body there are dozens of physical signs which could be elicited. Time prevents such an exercise and the 'basic' examination of the cardiovascular system should be limited to the essential physical signs which must be elicited in every case. These can be called 'first line physical signs' and will be dealt with in detail. When one of these signs is positive other physical signs may be elicited, complementing the finding. For example, when finding a wide pulse pressure (large difference between systolic and diastolic pressure) as in aortic incompetence, one must look for nailbed capillary pulsation. This sign would not normally be sought if there was a normal pulse pressure. Positive first line physical signs should trigger off an appropriate list of other physical signs which would confirm the suspicion of a diagnosis.

It is, therefore, mandatory to seek *while* examining not only for confirmatory physical signs but also for the significance of what is being elicited. It is not appropriate to 'add up' all your physical signs at the end of the examination and try and find a diagnosis. If the findings are analysed as the examination proceeds the correct diagnosis will be made before the end. It is important to have the patient lying comfortably and undressed enough to be able to see the chest and the abdomen fully as well as to be able to examine the legs. The examination of the patient can take place in any order one wishes but *Fig.* 3.1 is a useful reminder of what should be done.

General appearance

A quick look at the patient may give you a clue to the diagnosis.

1. Down's syndrome may be associated with a type of ventricular septal defect or patent ductus arteriosus.
2. Marfan's syndrome may be associated with aortic regurgitation.
3. Turner's syndrome may be associated with coarctation of the aorta.
4. Thyrotoxicosis may precipitate atrial fibrillation.
5. Myxoedema may cause a cardiomyopathy.
6. A malar flush can be present in mitral stenosis.

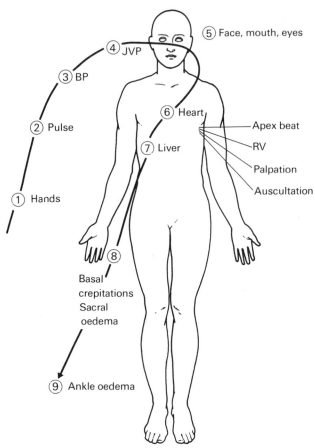

Fig. 3.1.   Suggested order for examining a 'cardiac' patient.

The hands

1.   *Temperature*

Poor left ventricular output will give cold extremities but care must be taken to remember local effects (e.g. cold room). The periphery may be cold due to Raynaud's phenomenon (often seen with beta-blockade), sweaty due to thyrotoxicosis and warm due to good peripheral perfusion. Carbon dioxide retention causes a warm periphery with bounding pulses, and anxiety results in cool hands with moist palms.

2.   *Finger clubbing*

Clubbing of the finger nails occurs when the angle of the pulp of the nail between the nail and flesh disappears (*Fig.* 3.2), the nail itself is more curved and the nailbed 'spongy' to compression.

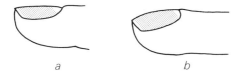

Fig. 3.2.   Showing (a) Normal finger-nail profile, (b) finger-clubbing.

Early clubbing is often difficult to see. Schamroth's sign is useful here (*Fig.* 3.3).

Finger clubbing may be due to:

Cardiac causes
1.   Bacterial endocarditis.
2.   Cyanotic congenital heart disease.
Respiratory causes
1.   Carcinoma of the bronchus.
2.   Chronic suppurative chest disease.
3.   Fibrosing alveolitis.
4.   Tuberculosis.
Others
1.   Congenital.
2.   Cirrhosis of the liver.
3.   Inflammatory bowel disease.

The cause of clubbing is unknown. It may also affect the toes.

3.   *Cyanosis*

The patient has a bluish colour which may range from barely dusky to navy blue. This may be central where the blood is not being oxygenated or peripheral where excessive oxygen is removed from the blood. Look at the tongue: it is blue in central cyanosis and pink in peripheral cyanosis. In both types the fingers, lips

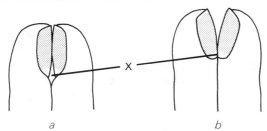

Fig. 3.3.   (a) Fingers held together – space seen at point 'X' as a result of normal angles in the fingers. (b) Positive Schamroth's sign. 'X' space is lost as a result of clubbing.

and feet will be dusky or blue. If you are uncertain if a patient's tongue is cyanosed compare it with a healthy nurse's.

4.   *Splinter haemorrhages*
Small linear haemorrhages may occur in both finger and toe nails due to local trauma. In the absence of trauma, subacute bacterial endocarditis (SBE) is a cause. If a patient is suspected of SBE, daily checks of the nails are necessary. The spontaneous appearance of new splinter haemorrhages can then be readily recorded and become highly significant.

5.   *Anaemia*
Pallor of the palmar creases indicates a marked level of anaemia, usually less than 6 g/dl.

6.   *Palmar erythema*
Erythema (redness) on the thenar and hypothenar eminences suggests liver impairment. Right heart failure congests the liver and impairs its function. In extreme cases liver cirrhosis may occur. Palmar erythema tends to be over-diagnosed.

The pulse
Several different pulses are examined and their presence or absence noted but more particularly their rate, rhythm, character and volume are determined. To do this first feel the radial pulse on one side and then simultaneously palpate the other radial, followed by femoral, carotid and possibly brachial pulses.

1.   *Rate*
Count the rate over 15 s. Avoid casual phrases such as 'the rate is somewhere around 100'. Bradycardia occurs with pulses < 60/min and tachycardia with > 100/min.

2.   *Rhythm*
The rhythm may be 'regular' (usually sinus rhythm but not always), 'regularly irregular' (sinus arrhythmia, regular ventricular ectopic beats) or 'irregularly irregular' (nearly always atrial fibrillation but can be sinus rhythm with ectopic beats). Sinus arrhythmia is common up to the age of 35–40 years.

3.   *Character and volume*
The normal pulse may be described as full. In left ventricular failure or shock from any cause the pulse is usually weak while in conditions with carbon dioxide retention the pulse is bounding (*Fig.* 3.4). In patients with aortic stenosis the restriction to flow imposed by the distorted valve causes a slow rising and plateau pulse in the presence of moderate to severe stenosis. This may be best felt over the carotid arteries.

A collapsing pulse is caused by a wide pulse pressure (*Fig.* 3.5) (a good guide is when the pulse pressure exceeds the diastolic pressure). This is typical of aortic incompetence but is very commonly caused in the elderly by arteriosclerosis (e.g. BP 190/90).

The pulse of hypertrophic cardiomyopathy is described as jerky, i.e. a normal pulse pressure with rapid rise and fall. A bisferiens pulse ('twice beating') occurs in moderate aortic stenosis with some regurgitation. If the radial pulse can be palpated 2–4 inches (5–10 cm) above the wrist, arteriosclerosis is nearly always present.

4.   *The normal pulse shape*

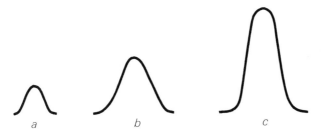

Fig. 3.4.   (a) Weak pulse in left ventricular failure or shock. (b) Normal pulse. (c) Bounding pulse in carbon dioxide retention or anaemia.

5.   *Abnormal pulses*

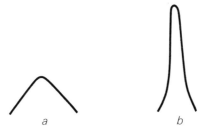

Fig. 3.5.   (a) Slow, rising pulse. (b) Collapsing pulse.

Check that both carotid vessels pulsate normally. Compare the radial pulse with the femoral pulse at the same time. Both of these pulses are approximately the same distance from the heart and in the presence of coarctation (narrowing) of the aorta the femoral artery pulsation will be delayed and weak. This is an important physical sign to look for, particularly in children.

Two variations of the force of the pulse are important:

a.   Pulsus 'paradoxus' (Fig. 3.6)

During inspiration the thorax takes in more blood and the pulmonary vascular bed expands slightly. There is a temporary diminution of blood being delivered to the left ventricle so that a small decrease in the pulse volume occurs during inspiration. This is not normally palpable but when extreme intrathoracic pressure changes occur, e.g. in asthma, the paradox may be quite marked.

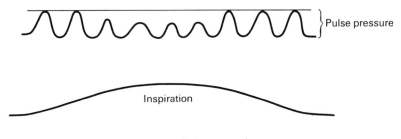

Pulse pressure

Inspiration

Fig. 3.6.   Pulsus paradoxus.

Strictly speaking it is not a paradox at all. Similarly, in constrictive pericarditis when filling of the heart is impaired, paradox may be demonstrated and is a most useful sign. A drop of more than 20 mmHg during inspiration would be regarded as 'pulsus paradoxus'.

b.   Pulsus alternans (Fig. 3.7)

Pulsus alternans occurs when consecutive beats show a difference greater than 20 mmHg systolic and the phenomenon is recurrent. The mechanism is not known and it is quite rare but when it does occur it is a bad prognostic sign.

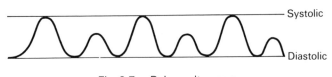

Systolic

Diastolic

Fig. 3.7.   Pulsus alternans.

Blood pressure

Good technique in measuring blood pressure is essential. The brachial artery should be at the level of the heart. The radial pulse should be palpated as the cuff is being inflated. In this way a reasonable idea of the systolic pressure is obtained before auscultating. The cuff is deflated gradually and the Korotkoff sounds listened for (*Fig.* 3.8). The appearance of the sounds reflects the systolic

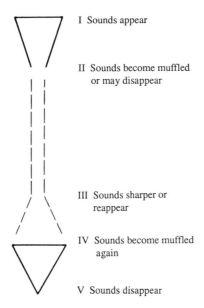

Fig. 3.8.   The Korotkoff sounds. I = systolic pressure. The period between II and III is called the auscultatory gap. True diastolic pressure lies between IV and V but nearer V.

pressure and the complete disappearance of sounds (not muffling of the sounds) is diastolic pressure. Occasionally the disappearance of sounds may not occur until 0 mmHg. This may be found in severe aortic regurgitation but more commonly if the subject is very anxious. If the disappearance of sounds (phase V) is more than 10 mmHg below the muffling of sounds (phase IV), the latter is a more accurate assessment of diastolic pressure.

When examining the patient take the blood pressure at the beginning and end of your examination. As the patient relaxes the systolic pressure may fall by as much as 80 mmHg. A large cuff is essential for fat arms as the readings may be falsely too high. The inflatable part of the cuff must cover at least half the circumference of the arm. If it does not a large cuff should be used.

In patients in whom dizziness is a significant symptom, lying and standing blood pressure should be taken and any postural drop noted.

If high blood pressure is suspected examination of the optic fundi must be performed, looking for signs of hypertensive retinopathy.

Occasionally there is a marked difference (>20 mmHg) in the blood pressure between the two arms. If this is the case it is usually due to atheroma and not a coarctation (narrowing) of the aorta which is a rare condition. About 25 per cent of the population will have a difference of 10 mmHg systolic between the two arms. This is a normal variation.

The jugular venous pulse

Eliciting this physical sign often causes much difficulty. Jugular venous pressure (JVP) is measured from observation of the internal jugular vein. It is not visible but acts as a pulsation manometer, the pulsations themselves being visible along the line of the vein which lies between the two heads of the sternomastoid muscle and the angle of the jaw. The easily seen external jugular vein is of limited value as it is often tortuous, kinked and contains valves.

Height

With the patient relaxed at approximately 45° the height of the JVP is taken from the sternal angle (roughly the position of the right atrium). Normal is up to 4–5 cm. Venous pressure falls on inspiration and rises on expiration. When the JVP is very high the ear lobes may waggle. Abdominal pressure over the liver (hepatojugular reflex) will increase the JVP in incipient heart failure but only by about 1 cm when the venous pressure is already raised. In normal patients abdominal pressure can cut off the venous return and reduce the JVP. In others it causes a transient rise in pressure which clears within a beat or two.

It is common, if the JVP is not seen to say 'the JVP is 0'. This is not true because the pressure may be anything from +5 to −5 cmH$_2$O. The correct description is 'the JVP is not raised'.

Wave form

This is best observed with the patient lying flat. Shining a torch across the neck may help view the pulsation, which should be timed by placing your thumb gently on the opposite carotid artery. An 'a' wave will occur just before the carotid pulsation. In the healthy person only the 'a' wave is normally visible.

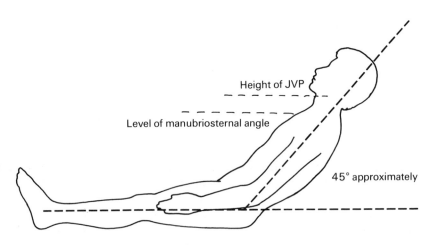

Height of JVP

Level of manubriosternal angle

45° approximately

Fig. 3.9.   Suggested position for examining the JVP.

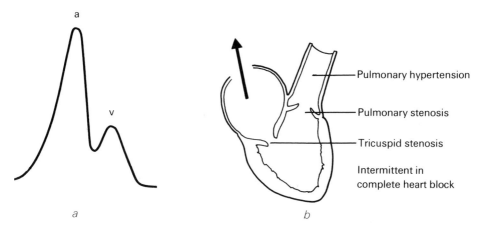

Fig. 3.10.   Large 'a' waves (a) and conditions causing them (b).

Clinically, observation must be made for abnormal or pathological 'a' or 'v' waves. Abnormal 'a' waves, occurring just before carotid pulsation are caused by pulmonary hypertension, pulmonary stenosis and rarely tricuspid stenosis. Abnormal 'v' waves occur coincident with carotid pulsation and are caused only by tricuspid regurgitation.

Cannon waves occur in complete heart block when the atrium contracts against a closed tricuspid valve. They are not true 'a' waves.

The neck

An enlargement of the thyroid gland (a goitre) may be obvious but its palpation from behind when the patient swallows is the only certain way of being sure it is the thyroid gland. If it is enlarged check for evidence of myxoedema or thyrotoxicosis. A bruit may be heard over the gland in advanced cases of thyrotoxicosis but this is now rare because thyrotoxicosis is usually diagnosed much earlier.

Both carotid vessels should be palpated and auscultated. A bruit over either vessel may be due to local atheroma or to the transmitted murmur of aortic stenosis.

The face

Look in the mouth at the tongue and mucous membranes for cyanosis. If it is present it represents a true lack of oxygenation (more than 5 g of reduced haemoglobin). The causes of cyanosis may be cardiac, respiratory or haematological in origin. Jaundice should be looked for in the sclerae and anaemia in the mucous membranes of the eyelid. If the mucous membranes are very pale the haemoglobin is usually less than 9 g/dl. If exophthalmos is present thyrotoxicosis should be considered.

Xanthelasma are seen in the palpebral fissure below the eye or just above it. They suggest hypercholesterolaemia but the cholesterol may be normal.

Xanthoma are cholesterol deposits seen on the tendons of the hand, over the elbows, and on the Achilles tendons. Hypertriglyceridaemia is occasionally seen as yellow deposits on the buttocks.

An arcus senilis is a white rim around the cornea which may suggest ischaemic heart disease if seen in a young patient, i.e. < 40 years. Mitral facies occurs with mitral valve disease when the cheeks become a dark red/blue colour but situated slightly higher over the malar bones than is generally seen with healthy 'rosy' cheeks.

The chest

Remembering the classic approach of observation, palpation, percussion and auscultation, in that order, is useful in examination of the heart because there is a tendency to rush to listen with the stethoscope.

Observation of the chest has probably already been done by this stage but certain points are important. Obvious pulsation in the chest may be the apex beat, right ventricle or a left ventricular aneurysm. If there is any deformity of the thoracic cage the heart may be slightly distorted and a murmur is common. Pectus excavatus, pigeon chest and kyphoscoliosis often result in an innocent systolic murmur.

Apex beat

Before the days of chest X-rays, long-term monitoring of the size of the heart could only be performed by carefully registering the most lateral and inferior part at which the left ventricle could be palpated. This is the apex beat.

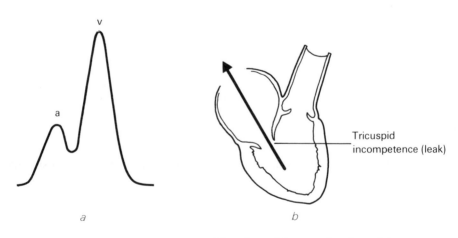

Fig. 3.11.   Large 'v' waves (a) and condition causing them (b).

When the position of the apex beat has been determined it is important next to decide upon its character. The normal apex beat (feel it on yourself but in the normal position for examining the cardiovascular system – 45° supine) is a single impulse which is relatively easy to feel but not excessively so. It is located in the fifth interspace in the mid-clavicular line. There are three abnormal apex beats of which it is useful to know the character.

1.   *Thrusting*
When the left ventricle is handling a larger volume of blood than normal (volume overload) such as occurs with mitral or aortic valve incompetence, the left ventricular cavity becomes dilated and the muscle very vigorous in its action. The apex beat is, therefore, felt over a large area (at least two finger-breadths) and is forceful and thrusting.

In a similar situation the apex beat may be felt over a large area but be rather weak, e.g. a cardiomyopathy.

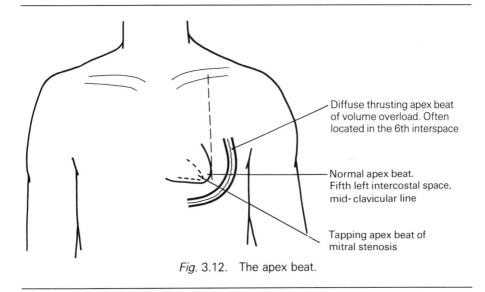

Diffuse thrusting apex beat of volume overload. Often located in the 6th interspace

Normal apex beat. Fifth left intercostal space, mid-clavicular line

Tapping apex beat of mitral stenosis

Fig. 3.12.   The apex beat.

2.   *Sustained*
In aortic stenosis or systemic hypertension there is left ventricular hypertrophy due to pressure overload. The apex beat thus becomes very forceful but over a small area and is not displaced. The chief characteristic is that it is sustained during systole.

3.   *Tapping*
When the mitral valve is stenosed the left ventricle receives less blood during diastole. The left ventricle becomes small and the apex beat is barely felt and is of brief duration. It is described as tapping.

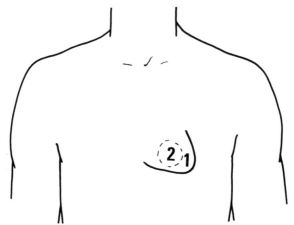

Fig. 3.13.   Double apex beat of a left ventricular aneurysm. Beats 1 and 2 are out of phase; 2 is the aneurysm, 1 is the apex beat.

When palpating the apex beat, a double impulse is occasionally felt. This may be due to a left ventricular aneurysm (*Fig.* 3.13).

The right ventricle

The right ventricle is only palpable if it is abnormal. An enlarged right ventricle causes heaving at the left sternal edge which is felt by placing the hand over this area. It is often better demonstrated if the fingers point laterally and can be seen to move (*Fig.* 3.14).

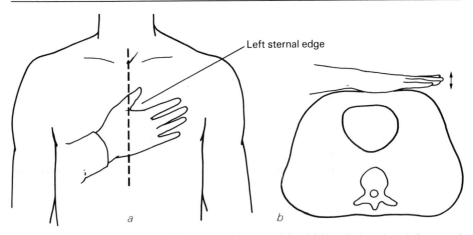

Fig. 3.14.   Palpation of abnormal right ventricle. (a) Hand placed on left sternal edge. (b) As the right ventricle heaves the tips of the fingers can be seen to move.

A right ventricular heave means increased right ventricular pressure which is almost always due to pulmonary hypertension. Occasionally it can be due to pulmonary stenosis or primary tricuspid incompetence as well as some forms of congenital heart disease.

Further palpation and auscultation

Palpation and then auscultation now proceed over the precordium in what are traditionally known as the mitral, aortic, tricuspid and pulmonary areas. This is misleading because the valves are not beneath the areas described, and in addition murmurs can be heard which are not necessarily associated with valve lesions. The 'traditional' sites are shown in *Fig.* 3.15 but ought to be slightly modified.

The precise characteristics of these murmurs will be dealt with in Chapter 6.

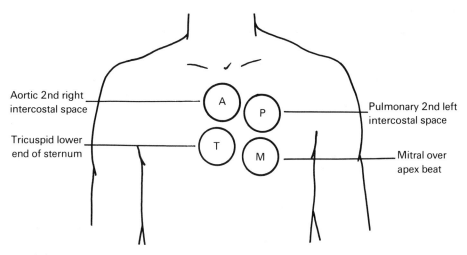

Aortic 2nd right intercostal space

Tricuspid lower end of sternum

Pulmonary 2nd left intercostal space

Mitral over apex beat

Fig. 3.15.   Surface points at which sounds and murmurs arising from the four heart valves are best heard.

In practice, therefore, both palpation and auscultation must be performed all over the precordium, i.e. over the aortic area and into the neck, the left sternal edge, the tricuspid and mitral areas, the axilla and the pulmonary area. After this procedure the patient should sit forward and breathe out to accentuate the murmur of aortic incompetence and lie on the left side to hear mitral stenosis better. Palpation is important for picking up thrills, i.e. palpable murmurs, although these are uncommon unless the turbulence is vigorous. They are most likely to occur with aortic stenosis or a ventricular septal defect but all murmurs can be accompanied by a thrill.

The aortic valve lies at the level of the third costal cartilages in the midline. The valve is situated in the outflow tract of the left ventricle which lies behind the right ventricle, i.e. the left ventricle is the posterior ventricle. The aorta itself arches forward, upwards and to the right before turning posteriorly leftwards and downwards. Aortic stenosis will, therefore, cause haemodynamic turbulence in the aorta, i.e. over the second right intercostal space and aortic incompetence will cause turbulence in the ventricle beneath the aortic valve in the third and fourth left intercostal spaces. Such is the vigorous nature of the turbulence of aortic stenosis that it is easily heard over the carotid arteries (*Fig.* 3.16).

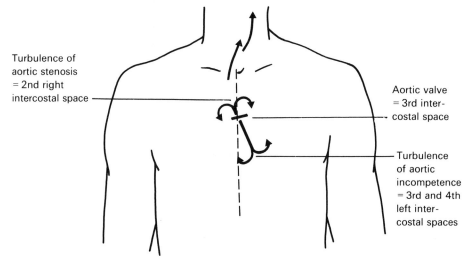

Turbulence of aortic stenosis = 2nd right intercostal space

Aortic valve = 3rd inter-costal space

Turbulence of aortic incompetence = 3rd and 4th left inter-costal spaces

Fig. 3.16.   Distribution of aortic valve sounds and murmurs.

Aortic incompetence is more easily heard with the patient leaning forward and breathing out.

The mitral valve is almost in the midline as well but a little lower than the aortic valve. It is angled towards the apex of the heart.

In mitral stenosis a jet of turbulent blood will strike the apex directly so that a diastolic murmur will be heard localized to the mitral area (*Fig.* 3.17). It is accentuated if the patient lies on his left side.

With mitral regurgitation vigorous turbulence occurs in the left atrium which acts as an echo chamber and transmits the murmur (which is pansystolic) widely over the precordium. Mitral regurgitation is thus heard over the mitral area, into the axilla and towards the midline (*Fig.* 3.18). As a rule the murmur is not conducted into the carotid arteries.

The pulmonary valve is in almost the same position as the aortic valve but faces the left shoulder. Pulmonary stenosis is thus heard over the traditional

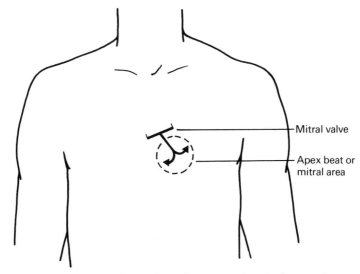

Fig. 3.17. Distribution of sounds and murmurs in mitral stenosis.

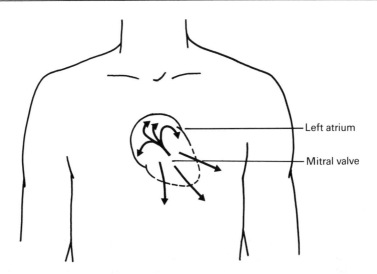

Fig. 3.18. Distribution of sounds and murmurs in mitral incompetence.

pulmonary area but pulmonary incompetence is heard along the right and left sternal edge (*Fig.* 3.19). It is often difficult to distinguish from the murmur of aortic incompetence but in aortic incompetence the pulse pressure is wide.

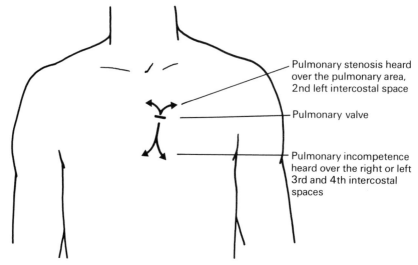

Fig. 3.19.   Distribution of sounds and murmurs in pulmonary valve disease.

The tricuspid valve lies in a similar position to the mitral valve but the turbulence which occurs with stenosis or incompetence of this valve is heard best towards the lower end of the sternum. The murmur of tricuspid stenosis is loudest over the traditional tricuspid area while tricuspid incompetence is heard widely over the tricuspid area and towards the apex (*Figs.* 3.20, 3.21).

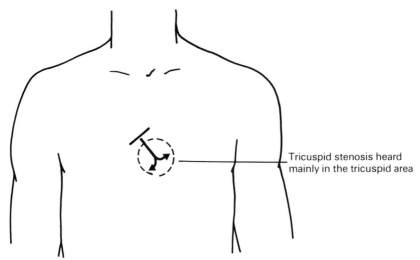

Fig. 3.20.   Distribution of sounds and murmurs in tricuspid stenosis.

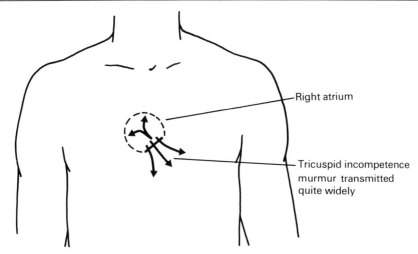

Fig. 3.21.   Distribution of sounds and murmurs in tricuspid incompetence.

The first heart sound is caused by sudden cessation of flow at the end of diastole when the A-V valves close. In the majority of patients it is split into its mitral and tricuspid components (M, T). In mitral stenosis when the cessation of flow is very abrupt the first heart sound is loud. In aortic stenosis and left bundle branch block a soft M is heard and it is variable in complete heart block and atrial fibrillation.

The second heart sound is caused by sudden cessation of flow at the end of systole when the aortic and pulmonary valves close (*Fig.* 3.22).

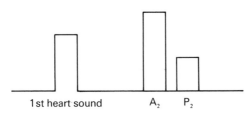

1st heart sound   A$_2$ P$_2$

Fig. 3.22.   The normal heart sounds.

When a person breathes in and out splitting of the second heart sound varies. On inspiration more blood is drawn into the thorax and on into the right ventricle. The time that the right ventricle takes to eject the blood is prolonged, and the second sound is split widely (especially well heard in children and young people). On expiration the right ventricular ejection time is shortened and the second heart sound is less split or not actually split at all (*Fig.* 3.23).

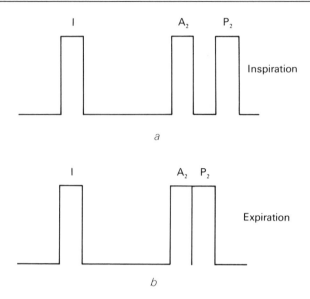

Fig. 3.23. Effect of (a) inspiration, (b) expiration on heart sounds.

In systemic hypertension the raised diastolic pressure causes more abrupt cessation of systolic flow and A_2 thus becomes louder. Similarly, pulmonary hypertension causes a louder P_2.

Wide splitting of the second heart sound may occur in an atrial septal defect (see Chapter 7) right bundle branch block, pulmonary stenosis and massive pulmonary embolism. Delay in the electrical activation of the right ventricle in right bundle branch block increases right ventricular ejection time and so P_2 is widely split from A_2.

Reversed splitting occurs in aortic stenosis and left bundle branch block (*Fig.* 3.24). In tight aortic stenosis the left ventricular ejection time may be so prolonged that A_2 occurs after P_2. During inspiration P_2 is prolonged and the second heart sound appears to be single (*Fig.* 3.25). In left bundle branch block the electrical delay in the left ventricle causes an increased left ventricular ejection time and so delays A_2. Note the paradoxical nature of the second sound in aortic stenosis or left bundle branch block. Two additional heart sounds are important: the third and fourth heart sounds.

The third heart sound is created by the rapid filling of the left ventricle. As blood suddenly enters from the atrium during early diastole it will cause a thud against the left ventricular wall. This is normal until the age of about 40 years but after that may represent heart failure. In mitral incompetence, much of the stroke volume will enter the left atrium so that a large quantity of blood will return to the left ventricle in early diastole. The blood 'thuds' against the ventricular wall and creates the third heart sound. In this case it does not

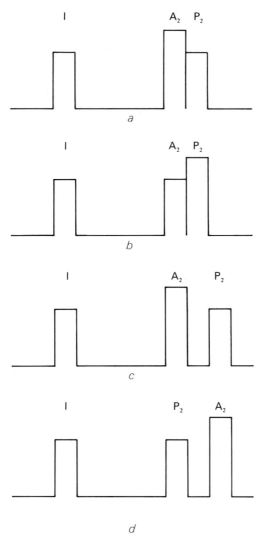

Fig. 3.24. Variations in the second heart sound. (a) Loud A_2 = systemic hypertension. (b) Loud P_2 = pulmonary hypertension. (c) Wide split second sound = ASD or RBBB. (d) Reversed split second sound = AS or LBBB.

necessarily represent heart failure but is an indication of the degree of mitral incompetence.

The fourth heart sound occurs when the atrium contracts against an already taut left ventricle. This event, occurring late in diastole, may cause another thud against the left ventricular wall. It may be heard in healthy hearts but when vigorous and loud usually represents heart failure (*Fig.* 3.26).

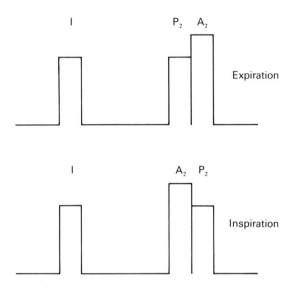

Fig. 3.25.   Reversed 'paradoxical' splitting of the second heart sound in LBBB or aortic stenosis.

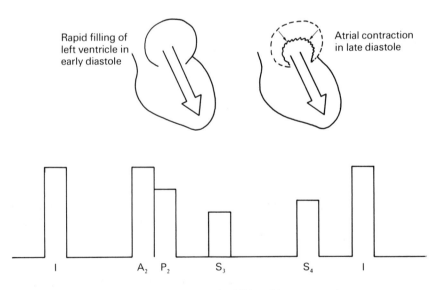

Fig. 3.26.   Generation of additional heart sounds.

With auscultation of the heart it is best to establish a routine for each examination. The following is the basic minimum that you should do every time you listen to a patient's heart.

1.   Auscultate in all areas with the patient lying comfortably, i.e.
    a. Aortic and carotid area
    b. Left and right sternal edges
    c. Pulmonary area
    d. Tricuspid area
    e. Mitral area and axilla
2.   Sit the patient forward and ask him to breathe out – listen for aortic incompetence.
3.   Lie the patient on the left side and listen for mitral stenosis and incompetence.
4.   Sum up your findings:
    a. Heart sounds one and two
    b. Added sounds, i.e. third and fourth heart sounds
    c. Murmurs, taking each one in turn and describing it accurately.

Other physical signs

Lung bases
Auscultation of the lung bases for evidence of pulmonary oedema is essential. As pulmonary oedema accumulates the alveoli are compressed and the air content inside them reduced. On taking a deep breath the alveoli crackle open giving a characteristic sound known as basal crepitations or crackles. In normal people a few alveoli will collapse while they are recumbent. Only if crepitations ('creps') persist after taking a good hearty cough are they significant. 'Innocent' crepitations will be cleared by coughing.

The liver
Right heart failure causes engorgement and thus enlargement of the liver. Palpation of the liver must be very careful in order to avoid possible confusion with other forms of liver disease. In right heart failure the liver will be:
1.   Enlarged.
2.   Tender.
3.   Smooth.
4.   If tricuspid incompetence is present it will pulsate. A large regurgitant jet of blood through the tricuspid valve will be transmitted to the liver. Care must be taken to check that it is actually the liver which is pulsating and not a transmitted pulsation from the abdominal aorta.

Oedema
Fluid retention is a common feature of congestive cardiac failure and when it develops in the tissues it will fall under the effect of gravity to the lowest part of the body. If the patient is walking or sitting most of the time the ankles will

swell, but if the patient is lying in bed oedema will appear predominantly over the sacral area. This is called 'dependent oedema'. Its major characteristic is that it is pitting. If a finger is pressed into the oedematous area a depression or pit will be temporarily created as the fluid is pushed out of the way. In long-standing oedema fibrosis may set in and pitting is no longer seen.

●   **Summary**

After history taking and examination a diagnosis should be sought. This is usually not too difficult but what is important is the severity of the lesion. With aortic stenosis, for example, the basic or anatomical diagnosis is straightforward enough but what functional effect is the narrowed valve having? In the cardiovascular system disease can have six major functional effects:

1.   Heart failure.
2.   Arrhythmias.
3.   Pulmonary hypertension.
4.   Cyanosis (associated with heart failure).
5.   Infective endocarditis.
6.   Systemic or pulmonary emboli.

In assessing a patient the initial diagnosis should be qualified by looking for evidence of any of these functional derangements. Aortic stenosis with heart failure is obviously quite different from the same lesion without heart failure.

Finally, it is very important to look for supporting or secondary physical signs which will support a diagnosis but which are not normally elicited in the routine cardiovascular examination. These will be considered in detail in the chapters dealing with individual diseases.

4

Investigation of heart disease

● **The electrocardiogram (ECG)**

Recording an ECG

There are four limb leads and a chest lead. The leads are labelled R arm, L arm, etc. and should be attached correctly using electrode jelly. The patient should be comfortable and relaxed, otherwise shaking will ruin the trace. With the dial at 0 and the paper running, the 1 mV marker is depressed. The height of 1 mV should be 10 small squares on the ECG paper and serves to standardize the tracing so that the size of the QRS complexes, etc. can be measured accurately.

After standardizing the tracing leads I, II, III, aVR, aVL and aVF are recorded (*Fig.* 4.1). This merely involves turning the dial on the ECG monitor and recording about five or six complexes of each lead. If a closer examination of the rhythm is necessary a longer strip of lead II is advisable.

Next the chest must be recorded ('V' leads) (*Fig.* 4.2). The standard positions must be used or small changes on the ECG may be incorrectly considered as significant.

The significance of the leads

The 'standard' leads (I, II, III, aVR, aVL, aVF) are recorded from the limb electrodes (*Fig.* 4.1).

All the 'standard' leads are in the vertical plane and in simple terms 'look at' different areas of the heart (*Fig.* 4.3). Thus leads II, III, aVF 'look at' the inferior surface of the heart; leads I, aVL 'look at' the anterolateral surface of the heart; lead aVR is not very helpful and looks at the top of the heart (*Fig.* 4.3). The chest leads are all in the horizontal plane and 'look at' the front or the anterior surface of the heart (*Figs.* 4.4, 4.5).

Therefore, in people sustaining heart attacks an anterior myocardial infarction shows changes in leads V1–6, and inferior infarction in leads II, III and aVF and a lateral infarction in leads I and aVL.

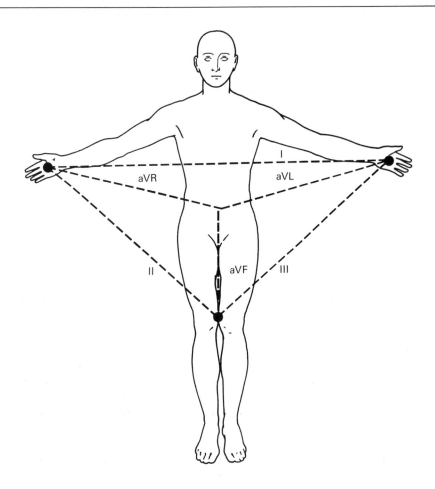

Fig. 4.1. Standard leads. aV = augmented voltage. R = right, L = left, F = foot.

The ECG complex

The wave form produced by the heart is conventionally labelled P, Q, R, S, T (*Figs.* 4.6, 4.7).

By convention any force moving towards an electrode is shown as a positive deflection, and any force moving away from an electrode is a negative deflection.

When depolarization occurs in the ventricle the spread of current follows a recognized path originating from the bundle of His (*Fig.* 4.8).

Depolarization first spreads across the septum away from the electrode causing a tiny Q wave. The electrocardiogram summates the forces in the ventricle which are thus towards the electrode causing a major positive R wave.

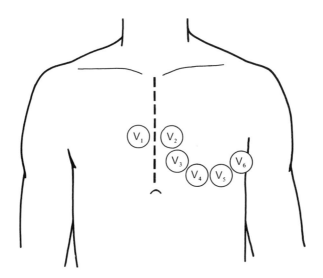

Fig. 4.2 Positions of the chest leads. V_1 = right sternal edge, 4th right intercostal space. V_2 = left sternal edge, 4th left intercostal space. V_3 = midway between V_2 and V_4. V_4 = midclavicular line, over apex beat. V_5 = same level as V_4, anterior axillary line. V_6 = same level as V_4, mid-axillary line.

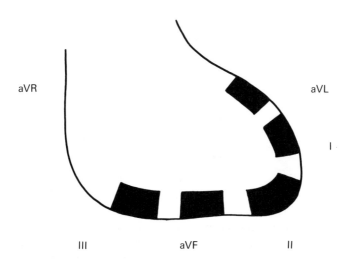

Fig. 4.3. Areas of the heart 'looked at' by the standard leads.

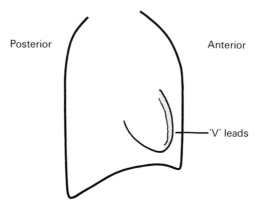

Fig. 4.4.   Area of the heart examined with the chest leads, viewed from the side.

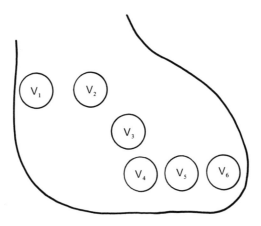

Fig. 4.5.   Area of the heart examined with the chest leads, viewed from the front.

The S wave is produced by late depolarization high in the ventricle going away from the electrode. The tiny Q wave seen in the normal ECG is physiological. Pathological Q waves represent dead myocardium which can produce no electrical current. In a myocardial infarction (*Fig.* 4.9) depolarization initially takes place across the intact septum. The right ventricular forces are dominant because of dead tissue in the left ventricle so the initial negative deflection becomes greater forming a pathological Q wave.

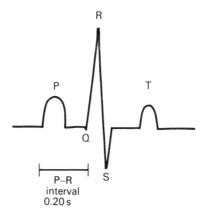

Fig. 4.6.   The normal electrocardiogram.

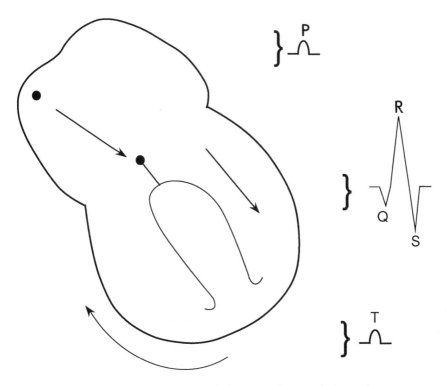

Fig. 4.7.   How the normal electrocardiogram is formed.

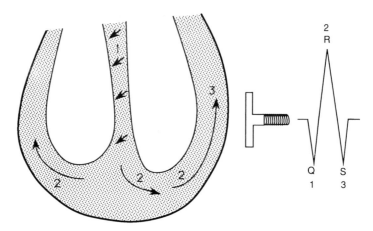

Fig. 4.8.   Sequence of electrical depolarization in normal ventricles and how it relates to the surface ECG.

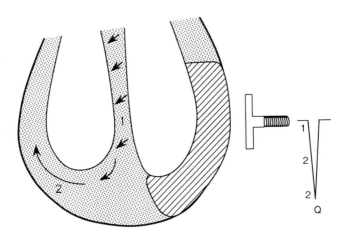

Fig. 4.9.   Sequence of electrical depolarization in an infarcted ventricle (striped segment) and how it relates to the surface ECG.

A pathological Q wave is greater than 0.04 (one small square) and more than one-third of the succeeding R wave.

The raised ST segment represents injured myocardium. A myocardial cell normally creates a resting potential inside itself of about −90 mV. An injured cell can only create a lower resting potential, say −40 mV.

● The chest radiograph (X-ray)

The correct name for the normal chest study is a 'PA' (posteroanterior) chest radiograph. This means that the anteriorly situated heart is as close to the film as possible and its image will be minimally enlarged (*Fig.* 4.10).

The chest radiograph is very important in cardiovascular disease. First the heart and then the lungs should be carefully observed.

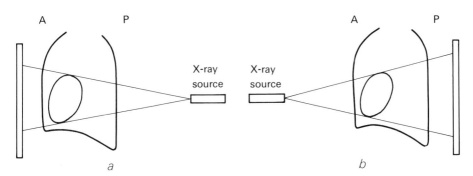

Fig. 4.10.   Cardiac radiography. (a) Normal PA X-ray. (b) AP X-ray (portable X-ray for patients in bed).

The size of the heart

The normal heart diameter is less than 50 per cent of the diameter of the chest. This is called the cardiothoracic ratio (CTR) (*Fig.* 4.11). If the heart is >50 per cent CTR it is enlarged and there is definitely some abnormality (except in neonates when the CTR is up to 60 per cent).

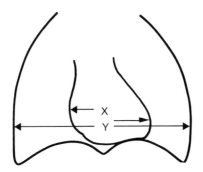

Fig. 4.11.   Cardiothoracic ratio (CTR). X = diameter of heart. Y = diameter of chest. X/Y = 50 per cent in normal hearts.

Chamber enlargement

It is very tempting to say that the left ventricle is enlarged if the cardiomegaly appears to be mostly to the left of the midline and conversely to say that there is right ventricular enlargement if the cardiomegaly is mostly to the right. This is a dangerous assumption and on a PA film the only chamber enlargement which can be seen for certain is the left atrium (*Fig.* 4.12).

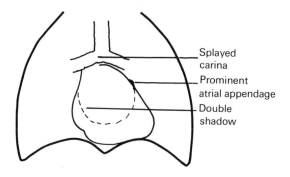

Splayed carina

Prominent atrial appendage

Double shadow

Fig. 4.12.   PA view showing left atrial enlargement.

A barium swallow helps to decide chamber enlargement because it outlines the posterior aspect of the heart. In addition the lateral views are more specific (*Fig.* 4.13).

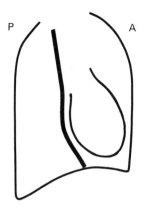

P   A

Fig. 4.13.   Lateral view in left atrial enlargement. The oesophagus is indented – normally it is straight.

Signs of heart failure

The radiological signs of heart failure are easily understood if you assume Hope's (1829) dam and stream theory as the cause of the problem, i.e. blood gets dammed back in the lungs because the heart is failing to pump it out. The signs which develop are therefore (*Fig.* 4.14):

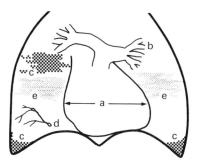

Fig. 4.14.   Radiological signs of heart failure (see text).

1. A large heart (**a**).
2. Increased upper lobe prominence of pulmonary arteries which are normally virtually empty of blood (**b**).
3. Signs of fluid outside the lungs (**c**)
    – in the fissures,
    – as small pleural effusions.
4. Signs of removal of that fluid, i.e. prominent lymphatic channels – Kerley B lines (**d**).
5. Fluid in the interstitial parts of the lungs (**e**).

Other important signs

Calcification may be seen in the valves (rheumatic heart disease) or in the pericardium (constrictive pericarditis) but is probably more often seen nowadays in aortic stenosis. An abnormal bulge on the left heart border may represent a left ventricular aneurysm. In congenital heart disease the aortic arch should be sought on the left (small in atrial septal defects and right sided in some cases of Fallot's tetralogy) and the presence of the major pulmonary arteries determined. Notching of the underside of the ribs occurs in coarctation of the aorta (above the age of 4 years).

● **Echocardiogram (echo)**

Ultrasound waves bounce off the different surfaces of the heart to form a moving picture of the various chambers and vessels. The waves (2.25–6 mHz) reflect from any fluid/solid interface and are recorded usually from the 4th left intercostal space. Lung tissue scatters the ultrasound so that no recording can be made. The transducer both emits and receives the waves and information can be gathered on both structural and functional aspects of the heart (*Fig.* 4.15).

The echo is non-invasive, cheap and repeatable and can, therefore, be used to follow patients and observe changes.

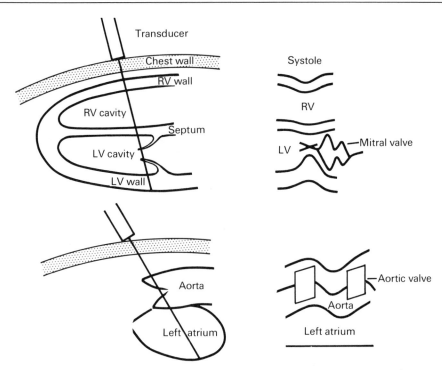

Fig. 4.15.   Echocardiography of the heart.

Structural changes

In paediatric cardiology congenital abnormalities such as a single ventricle can be seen easily and are increasingly obviating the need for cardiac catheterization.

In the adult chamber size is very important. A large dilated left ventricle may be typical of a congestive cardiomyopathy while a huge dilated left atrium may suggest mitral valve disease. Thickened, relatively immobile cusps of the mitral valve are easy to see in mitral stenosis and the diagnosis can be readily made. A pericardial effusion can be seen creating an echo-free space outside the heart and the echo is by far the best investigation for the condition.

Many other abnormalities of the heart can be diagnosed by echocardiography and for further information a larger textbook must be consulted.

Functional changes

Some assessment of the function of the left ventricle can be made by noting the degree of contraction of the ventricle.

This used to be fairly unreliable with the older echo techniques but modern two-dimensional (2-D) echocardiography (*Figs.* 4.16, 4.17) now gives a

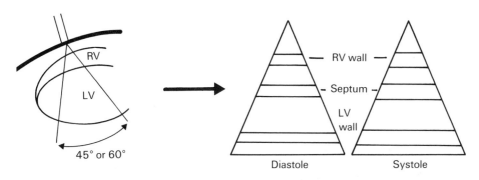

Fig. 4.16.   Diagram of two-dimensional (2-D) echocardiogram.

clear idea of left ventricular function in suitable echo patients. It is not, however, possible to get good echocardiographic data in all subjects, e.g. too obese, presence of chronic obstructive airways disease, etc. Using 2-D echo good estimates of cardiac output can also be obtained especially since the arrival of Doppler echocardiography. The latest techniques involve transforming the flow data into colour signals so that the operator can detect leaks, e.g. mitral incompetence, by means of detecting the changed colour.

Cardiac catheterization

A soft catheter introduced via a vein or artery can be passed into the great vessels and heart without too much difficulty. The brachial or femoral vessels are usually used and the vessels either exposed (brachial) or punctured by a needle (femoral). A venous catheter can successively reach the vena cava, right atrium, right ventricle, pulmonary artery and the peripheral lung vessels. An arterial catheter can reach the aorta and left ventricle and if carefully adapted can be introduced into the mouth of the coronary arteries. The left atrium in adults is usually reached directly by a trans-septal catheter. In this procedure a long wire from the femoral vein pierces the interatrial septum and a catheter is introduced over it and fed directly into the left atrium. These catheters provide four major types of information.

Pressure measurements

Manometer measurements via the catheters can be made in all chambers. This is very useful in determining valvular stenosis, e.g. in aortic stenosis the peak left

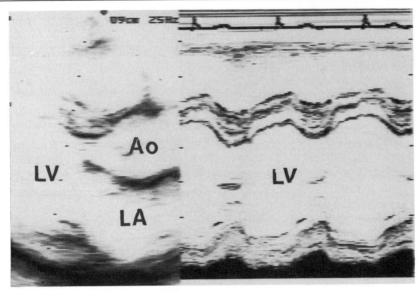

Fig. 4.17.   (a) 2-D echocardiogram of normal left ventricle (LV), left atrium (LA) and aorta (Ao). On the right is an M-mode trace of LV for comparison.

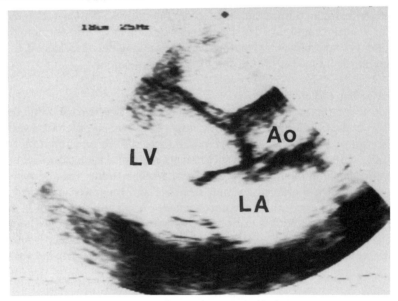

Fig. 4.17.   (b) 2-D echocardiogram of dilated LV. Note the different scale from the normal recording.

ventricular pressure will be much higher than the peak aortic pressure. The difference in pressures is known as the valve gradient (*Fig.* 4.18).

Another important pressure measurement is the left ventricular end diastolic pressure. A figure greater than 12 mmHg suggests a poorly contracting left ventricle.

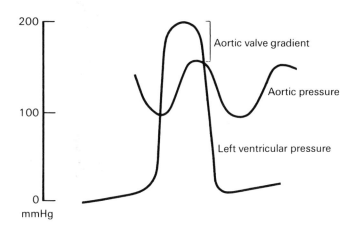

Fig. 4.18.   Pressure measurements in aortic stenosis.

Oxygen saturation measurements

If there is a connection between the two sides of the heart blood will be shunted from left to right in the early stages of life. Much later, when the pulmonary artery pressure reaches systemic levels blood will be shunted from right to left. The latter is obvious, the patient is blue (cyanosed), but the former needs documenting so that the degree of shunting can be measured. When the pulmonary flow exceeds the systemic flow by more than 2:1 an operation is usually indicated.

Oxygen saturations assess the degree of shunting as well as determining its site. When there is a sudden step up in oxygen levels a shunt must be present. The amount of step up is used to calculate the degree of shunting.

Cine angiography

The rapid injection of radio-opaque contrast medium (e.g. Lopamidol 370) enables the chambers of the heart to be seen quite accurately. The commonest use of this procedure in the adult is to outline the aorta or left ventricle. Any regurgitation through the aortic or mitral valve can be seen as the dye is pumped by the heart into the wrong chamber.

Angiography in children can be very useful in defining the precise nature and relationship of major vessels and chambers of the heart.

Coronary angiography

Specially shaped cardiac catheters can be relatively easily introduced into the coronary vessels from either the brachial artery (Sones technique) or the femoral artery (Judkins) (*Fig.* 4.19). About 5–10 ml of dye are rapidly injected to outline the arterial tree while a cine film is being taken. Views of the same coronary artery are taken from different angles using repeated injections of dye.

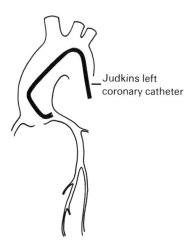

Judkins left coronary catheter

Fig. 4.19.   Coronary angiography.

The value of this technique is to assess the anatomy and any narrowing of the coronary arteries.

● Myocardial imaging using radioactive isotopes

Ischaemia and infarction of the myocardium can be detected using radioisotopes and a gamma camera.

Thallium-201

This isotope is taken up by the myocardium in proportion to its blood flow. The patient is exercised on a treadmill or bicycle and then at the peak of exercise the thallium is injected intravenously. The beauty of this technique is that for about 1 hour after injection the radioactivity from the heart still reflects the blood flow at the time of exercise. In this way good, relatively stable myocardial images can be obtained. Areas of large flow are 'hot' and areas of low flow, or ischaemia, are 'cold'.

After a further few hours the thallium redistributes to areas that are no longer ischaemic under resting conditions (as opposed to exercise) and the radioisotope image obtained is called a reperfusion scan. Thus one single injection of thallium will give both an exercise and a resting image of myocardial blood flow and reversible myocardial ischaemia can be assessed.

Technetium-99 – labelled pyrophosphate

This isotope is taken up by infarcted myocardial tissue and, therefore, a 'hot' spot represents ischaemic tissue – the opposite of the thallium scan.

This label is of greater use in assessing myocardial function. Red cells are labelled with it and then injected into the circulation to form a 'pool' of radioactive cells. By counting radioactivity over the heart a cine picture can be built up showing myocardial contraction in systole and relaxation in diastole. This is the gated blood pool scan (MUGA) and is a useful non-invasive way of assessing ejection fraction (how much blood is gated with each systole) and to a lesser extent ventricular wall motion (e.g. detecting aneurysms of the left ventricle). In congenital heart disease the isotope can be followed as it passes round the circulation and abnormal routes can be detected, e.g. transposition of the great arteries.

● Phonocardiography

Heart sounds, added sounds and murmurs can be recorded on paper using a small microphone on the chest. It is not an alternative to a cardiologist but can be used for timing sounds and murmurs and thereby assessing their significance.

● Apex cardiography

The pulse wave of the apex beat can be recorded with a variety of transducers. There is a similarity between the shape of the apex cardiogram and the left ventricular pressure and it is tempting to use it as a measure of left ventricular function. Its value is predominantly in research.

● Pulse wave recording and systolic time intervals

The shape and size of the pulse wave is recorded similarly to the apex cardiogram. A slow rising pulse of aortic stenosis (upstroke $> 0.22 \text{s}$) or a collapsing pulse of aortic incompetence can be clearly shown but digital assessment is often sufficient. Timing the various events in relation to the ECG may give an indication of left ventricular function (systolic time intervals). The great advantage is that it is non-invasive. It tends to be rather inaccurate however.

● Intracardiac electrophysiology

The technique of intracardiac electrophysiology is used to investigate rhythm disturbances and conduction defects. A number of pacing and/or recording electrodes are placed in various chambers and positions in the heart and the passage of either naturally arising or paced impulses can be followed. It is particularly useful for detecting otherwise hidden disease of the conducting system (such as sick sinus syndrome) or bypass tracts (such as in the Wolff–Parkinson–White syndrome). Recordings can be made from the bundle of His and the technique has also been called His bundle electrocardiography.

● Computed tomography and magnetic resonance scans

These highly specialized scanning techniques have been less useful in investigating heart disease because of the heart's mobility. They can be extremely useful for looking at aortic dissections, mediastinal swellings, etc. Undoubtedly they will have a major role to play in cardiac investigation in the future.

5

Practical and therapeutic procedures

● Cardiac resuscitation

One of the most frightening events in a student or houseman's career is having to deal with a cardiac arrest. In the hubbub which follows an arrest it is often difficult to do anything effectively and only after a lot of experience does one become 'comfortable' at an arrest. Treatment of cardiac arrest should always be carried out efficiently and enthusiastically. Every half-hearted attempt at resuscitation reduces the effectiveness of the team and its routine. Needless to say when a patient collapses unexpectedly from an unknown cause, resuscitation should be applied until all doubt is removed. It is desirable that when a patient is admitted who is liable to have a cardiac arrest, definite instructions are given to the nursing staff as to whether resuscitation should be attempted or not.

'Circulatory arrest' may not be cardiac in origin. It may be due to sudden blood loss or a simple faint. It is worth looking at the neck veins carefully. If they are engorged then circulatory arrest from a central cause is likely (exclude tension pneumothorax). If the neck veins are collapsed, bleeding or a faint are possibilities.

If a patient is likely to have a cardiac arrest prevention may be helped bearing in mind the following points:
1. Relieve fear and pain
2. Avoid hypotension
3. Watch the PO_2, pH, serum K^+ and urinary output
4. Monitor the ECG
5. Avoid urinary retention.

In addition, make sure the patient is on a hard bed and that the head of the bed can be removed if necessary.

Immediate management by ward staff

The classic signs of cardiac arrest are:
1. Unconsciousness
2. Absence of spontaneous respiration (sometimes agonal deep respiration is present)

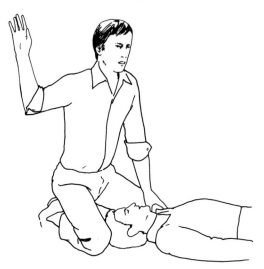

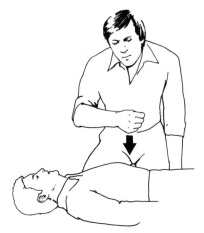

Fig. 5.1.   Call to someone to summon Cardiac Arrest Team.

Fig. 5.2.   Thump chest hard. This may restart the heart.

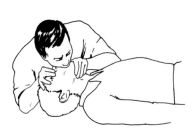

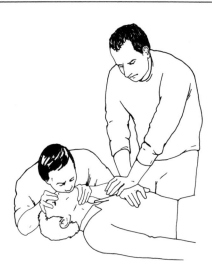

Fig. 5.3. Start mouth-to-mouth resuscitation after clearing airway. Watch rise and fall of chest.

Fig. 5.4.   Second person begins cardiac massage. Alternate massage and ventilation (five massages and one ventilation). This can all be done by one person if necessary.

3.   Absent pulses and heart sounds
4.   Dilated pupils
The first person at a cardiac arrest must begin resuscitation. There is no time for the person discovering the cardiac arrest to telephone. This must be done by someone else, even an ambulant patient.
1.   Call someone to dial the Cardiac Arrest Team (*Fig.* 5.1).
2.   Look for airways obstruction. Remove pillows, clear pharynx of food, vomit, foreign bodies and false teeth by hand if necessary. Hold the chin up and deliver a sharp blow to the patient's chest. This may restart normal cardiac rhythm (*Fig.* 5.2).
3.   Institute mouth-to-mouth resuscitation. This can be done by direct contact (with an intervening gauze if necessary) or a Brooke airway. Occlude the nose while you are doing this (*Fig.* 5.3).
4.   The second person should start cardiac massage. The heel of one hand is placed over the lower third of the sternum with the other hand on top. The sternum should be compressed 1½–2 inches (4–5 cm) with each compression. The optimum pressure is to 80 to 100 lb (36 to 45 kg) which can be achieved by the weight of the upper half of the body. Massage is more effective and less tiring if the arms are kept straight. The sternum should be compressed 80 times per minute. Massaging and ventilation must be applied alternately – five compressisons alternating with one inflation of the chest. If the patient is lying on a soft bed put a board under him (*Fig.* 5.4).
The above procedure of massage and ventilation will keep a patient in a reasonable condition for up to 1 hour.

Errors which prevent effective ventilation
1.   Not clearing the upper air passages of vomit, food or secretions.
2.   Wasting time with methodical aspiration during the immediate phase of treatment.
3.   Not hyperextending the neck adequately with the tongue clear of the pharynx.
4.   Not occluding the nose during mouth-to-mouth resuscitation.
5.   Not using a properly fitting mask when using an Ambu bag.
6.   Wasting time attempting to pass an endotracheal tube when unfamiliar with the technique.
7.   Not confirming adequate ventilation by watching the chest during mouth-to-mouth respiration.

Errors which prevent effective cardiac massage
1.   Insufficient pressure to really compress the heart between the sternum and spinal column.
2.   Massaging too fast.
3.   Not releasing the pressure on the chest completely after each compression thus preventing cardiac filling.

4.   Not having the hands placed in the proper position.
5.   Applying too much pressure to the chest and fracturing ribs, particularly in the elderly. Broken ribs, laceration of the lungs, liver, spleen and pericardium, fat or bone marrow embolism or rupture of major blood vessels should all be avoidable by good technique.

Arrival of the cardiac arrest team
Once the medical team has arrived the senior doctor must take charge. He must remain free to direct operations.

1.   *Ventilation*
Initially mouth-to-mouth resuscitation can be replaced by using an Ambu bag with an airway in the patient's mouth. Oxygen should be attached to this at 15 litres/minute.
As soon as the anaesthetist arrives endotracheal intubation is performed. This must be done by the anaesthetist or other experienced person or long delays will occur when the patient has no ventilation or output. The anaesthetist will probably need suction apparatus and this must be to hand as quickly as possible.

2.   *Establishing an intravenous line*
Sodium bicarbonate 4.2 per cent should be infused as quickly as possible. A saphenous vein cut-down at the ankle or using the jugular veins which are usually very prominent at a cardiac arrest is preferable to a prolonged search for an arm vein. Always give 10 ml calcium chloride or calcium gluconate straight away whatever the cause of the cardiac arrest. It will never do any harm and it may help myocardial contraction. Remember that calcium salts become insoluble calcium bicarbonate if injected into the sodium bicarbonate bottle. Therefore, give calcium as a bolus.
Once the patient has been resuscitated, change the bicarbonate to 5 per cent dextrose (not saline) until arterial pH is obtained.

3.   *Correcting acidosis*
Severe metabolic acidosis develops almost immediately after the onset of a cardiac arrest. The acidosis continues despite cardiac massage and ventilation; 200 ml of 4.2 per cent sodium bicarbonate (100 mEq) should be given immediately, followed by 100 ml every 5 minutes until the cardiac output is once again adequate.

4.   *The electrocardiogram*
The heart rhythm must be identified as early as possible. The majority of patients will be in ventricular fibrillation (VF) or asystole. Make sure the electrode plates are properly attached so that asystole does not look like VF. Suspend cardiac massage periodically so that a rhythm may be identified. A few patients may be in ventricular tachycardia or complete heart block.

Treatment

1.   *Ventricular fibrillation (VF)*

Electrical defibrillation (*Fig.* 5.5) is necessary but it is important to get the patient's myocardium as well oxygenated as possible before delivering the shock. Ventilation and massage must be continued until the moment before the shock. Everyone associated with cardiac arrests must be able to work the defibrillator.

a.   Put plenty of electrode jelly on the skin to avoid burns.

b.   Do not have a continuous smear of jelly between the electrodes or you will get a short circuit.

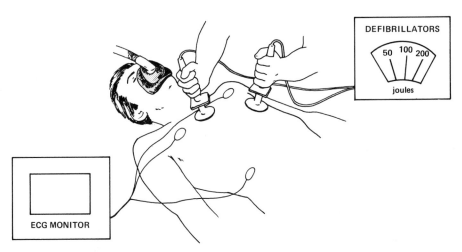

Fig. 5.5.   Technique of cardiac defibrillation.

c.   Make sure the shock is not 'synchronized' or the machine will never deliver the shock.

d.   Press on the paddles or you may not make contact.

e.   Stand clear of the bed and make sure everyone else does and that there is no direct physical contact with the patient other than with the defibrillator electrodes.

f.   Continue massaging the heart after the shock if no acceptable rhythm is produced.

g.   If an ordinary ECG machine or pacemaker is attached to the patient disconnect it before you defibrillate or you may damage the machine.

2.   *Asystole*

a.   Inject 5 ml of 1:10 000 adrenaline intravenously (i.v.).

b.   Inject 100 μg isoprenaline i.v.

3. *Ventricular tachycardia*

'Synchronized' DC shock is necessary (see Cardioversion, below). If the patient is conscious 10 mg diazepam i.v. may be necessary.

4. *Complete heart block*

a. Isoprenaline 5 mg in 500 ml run at 10–15 drops per minute may increase the ventricular rate.

b. A temporary pacemaker may need to be inserted by someone experienced in this technique.

5. *Other arrhythmias*

See chapter 9.

● **Cardioversion**

Tachyarrhythmias which are either life threatening (e.g. ventricular tachycardia) or causing a low output syndrome may need to be terminated by an electric shock. Medical treatment may be appropriate initially but cardioversion should be performed if an emergency develops. The principle is to deliver a high energy, short duration pulse of electricity to the heart which will leave long enough time following it for the sinus mode to take over as the heart's pacemaker.

Arrhythmias requiring cardioversion

1. Asynchronized – ventricular fibrillation.
2. Synchronized – supraventricular tachycardia; atrial fibrillation; other rapid atrial tachycardia; ventricular tachycardia.

Procedure

The patient is anaesthetized because a shock will cause intense spasm and pain in the chest wall and pectoral muscles. A light anaesthetic is all that is necessary and intravenous diazepam is also often sufficient. The patient only needs to be anaesthetized for a few minutes and an endotracheal tube is seldom necessary. Elective cardioversions are usually done as day cases and the patient is fit enough to go home the same evening although he should not be allowed to drive.

In converting some arrhythmias (particularly atrial fibrillation) to sinus rhythm there is a small but definite risk of systemic emboli. If the cardioversion is elective, anticoagulation with warfarin for 3 to 6 weeks beforehand is required. This is particularly the case if mitral valve disease has precipitated the atrial fibrillation. Anticoagulation should be continued subsequently until a particular rhythm (hopefully sinus) is definitely established. Changing rhythms could lead to systemic emboli.

There is little evidence that sinus rhythm will be maintained by using long-term anti-arrhythmic therapy following cardioversion. It may be important in a particular case but not as a routine. This situation may well change in the future with the arrival of newer more effective anti-arrhythmic agents.

Cardiac enzymes will rise a little after a cardioversion. This is presumably damage caused by the myocardial contraction but does not represent myocardial infarction.

● **Pacemaker insertion**

A pacemaker is an instrument designed to deliver a small electric current to the right ventricle in order to make the ventricles contract. Its prime use is in periods of very slow pulse when it will bring the heart rate back to a normal level. Pacemakers have also been used to terminate tachyarrhythmias but their use here is rare, i.e. antitachycardia pacemakers.

Indications
1.   Complete heart block
2.   The bradycardia of the sick sinus syndrome.

Both these arrhythmias may be associated with Stokes–Adams attacks and low output syndrome.

Complete heart block may be temporary or permanent. The sick sinus syndrome is usually permanent. It is important, therefore, to be able to pace a patient both temporarily and permanently.

Complete heart block not infrequently occurs with acute inferior myocardial infarction and may last for a few days. This patient needs a temporary pacemaker. However, permanent complete heart block is caused in the majority of cases by fibrosis and degeneration of the conducting tissue and so is not reversible and permanent pacing is required.

Complete heart block may be preceded by lesser degrees of conduction abnormality such as second degree heart block or bundle branch block (see chapter 9).

If the ECG shows right bundle branch block and either left anterior hemiblock (extreme left axis deviation $> -30°$) or left posterior hemiblock (extreme right axis deviation $> +120°$) there is a risk of complete heart block developing. If such a situation develops during a myocardial infarction a temporary pacemaker is required but if this is found by chance on an ECG with no immediate pathology, a permanent pacemaker is only required if the patient has dizzy spells or Stokes–Adams attacks, although this is still controversial.

After the temporary electrode is inserted it is passed on towards the apex of the right ventricle and then connected to a voltage source (see *Fig.* 5.6).

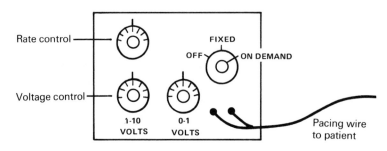

Fig. 5.6.   Typical external pacing 'box'.

Permanent pacing

The principles of insertion of a permanent pacemaker are the same as for a temporary pacemaker.

The permanent pacing box must be inserted under the skin and subcutaneous fat (*Fig.* 5.7). It is usually placed on top of the pectoralis major muscle but not in a position to interfere with shoulder movement. It is often preferable to have the permanent box on the left side if the patient is right handed so as to interfere with movement (e.g. a golf swing) as little as possible. The life of a pacemaker box varies according to its batteries. The lithium batteries currently used last 6 to 7 years or longer and are ideal in the majority of cases. When the batteries are losing power the rate may change a little and the wave impulse varies. The patient, therefore, must attend an outpatient clinic regularly for a pacemaker box checkup. When a change is necessary a new box is inserted and attached to the old pacemaker wire.

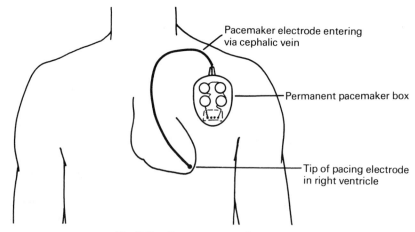

Fig. 5.7.   Permanent pacing system.

Complications
1.   The pacing wire may fall out of position (displaced).
2.   The pacing wire may penetrate the myocardium, increasing the threshold and stimulating the diaphragm.
3.   The threshold may exceed the output of the box despite an initially low threshold.
4.   Infection at the box site may occur.
5.   Rarely axillary vein thrombosis may develop.
6.   Excessively rarely, the pacing box fails or the pacing wire breaks.

Overall permanent pacing is one of the most cost-effective things we do in medicine and can transform the quality of life in those receiving them, e.g. people with frequent Stokes–Adams attacks.

● Pericardiocentesis

If fluid collects between the pericardium and myocardium (a pericardial effusion) drainage may be necessary. This may be desperately urgent (cardiac tamponade caused by a traumatic haemopericardium), moderately urgent (cardiac embarrassment caused by a large pericardial effusion) or an elective procedure in order to diagnose the cause of the pericardial effusion, e.g. malignant spread from adjacent structures.

The diagnosis can be made clinically if tamponade is present but if there is time an echocardiogram provides a clear answer. If the effusion is greater than 1 cm anteriorly pericardiocentesis is a reasonably safe procedure. Introducing a needle so close to the heart can be dangerous so the procedure must be done by an experienced doctor and where cardiac resuscitation can take place.

● Intra-aortic balloon pumping

When severe left ventricular failure develops from whatever cause, reducing the work load and increasing the coronary artery blood flow may improve the ventricle long enough for either natural or surgical improvement to take place. This can be achieved by inserting a balloon catheter into the lower thoracic aorta from the femoral artery. The balloon is designed to inflate during diastole and so raise the diastolic pressure and increase coronary flow. In systole the balloon collapses and reduces the afterload on the heart. The balloon catheter is triggered by the patient's ECG and can be extremely effective in increasing cardiac output (*Fig. 5.8*).

Intra-aortic balloon catheters should only be used if some recovery of the ventricle can be expected. It is not suitable for the patient who has had several massive myocardial infarctions because as soon as the balloon pump is switched off the patient will go downhill and die.

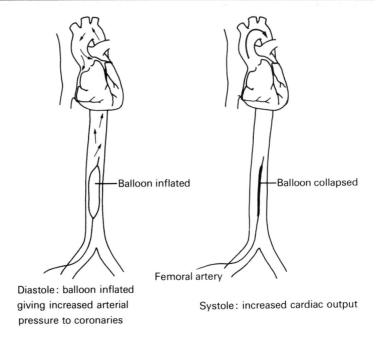

Diastole: balloon inflated
giving increased arterial
pressure to coronaries

Systole: increased cardiac output

Fig. 5.8.   Intra-aortic balloon counterpulsation.

It is very suitable for the postoperative cardiac surgery patient where poor left ventricular function may be purely temporary or a myocardial infarction patient who has a ruptured mitral valve or interventricular septum and in whom a valve replacement or septal repair operation would be possible. It is also used in pre-infarction angina where there is poor left ventricular function that is thought to be potentially salvageable.

6

Valvular heart disease

In valvular heart disease the valves may become stenosed, incompetent or a combination of the two. Although there are a number of causes only a few are common.

1. Rheumatic fever

As social standards have improved the incidence of rheumatic fever has dropped considerably. At the turn of the century the incidence of rheumatic heart disease was probably 200 times its present level. It is still very common, however, in Third World countries. Rheumatic fever occurs primarily in children (but ages range from 2 to 30 years) and begins with a β-haemolytic streptococcal sore throat. About 3 weeks after the sore throat the signs and symptoms of rheumatic fever begin with pyrexia, malaise, flitting joint pains (sometimes wrongly thought of as 'growing pains'), erythema marginatum, subcutaneous nodules and evidence of carditis. There appears to be an antigen–antibody response to the *Streptococcus* which results in rheumatic fever. The characteristic lesion is a perivascular granulomatous reaction and vasculitis – the Aschoff body. As there are no direct blood tests for rheumatic fever the diagnosis is made on clinical grounds using the modified Jones criteria.

Major	*Minor*
Polyarthritis	Fever
Carditis	Raised ASO titre
Erythema marginatum	Abdominal pain
Sydenham's chorea	Malaise
Subcutaneous nodules	Raised WCC or ESR
	Prolonged PR interval on the ECG

The diagnosis is considered positive if two major or one major and two minor criteria are found. A raised ASO titre (>250) only suggests a recent streptococcal infection.

The diagnosis is often very difficult to make in developed countries as many of the cases are very mild.

The characteristic of the arthritis is that one day a joint, e.g. the knee, may be red, swollen and painful and the next day completely normal while another joint, e.g. the elbow, may flare up in the interim. Sydenham's chorea consists of jerky facial or limb movements which occur spontaneously and are worse if the patient is nervous but which disappear during sleep. These children used to be thought to be 'putting it on' until the diagnosis was made. Pericarditis, myocarditis and endocarditis occur in rheumatic fever although only the last usually causes problems. Initially, oedema of the valves causes murmurs but later fusion of the cusps, destruction of the cusps or rupturing of the chordae tendinae seriously damage the valves (*Fig.* 6.1).

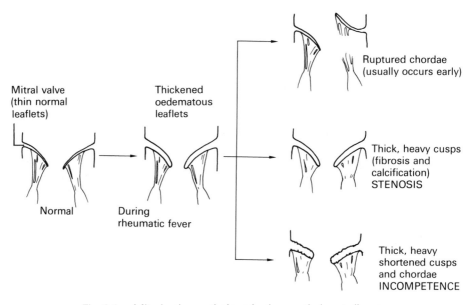

Fig. 6.1.   Mitral valve pathology in rheumatic heart disease.

In stenosis of the valve there is often fusion of the edges of the cusps narrowing the orifice and giving a 'fish mouth' effect to the valve which can sometimes be seen with two-dimensional echocardiography (*Fig.* 6.2).

Although carditis may exist during the episode of rheumatic fever it is often years before damage and destruction result in failure of the heart. In Third World countries where children may get the illness every year, valve replacements are often performed in teenagers.

Only about 50–60 per cent of those patients who contract rheumatic fever develop carditis and the only treatment for the acute illness is bed-rest and aspirin. Prednisolone has been used but there is no evidence that it is superior to

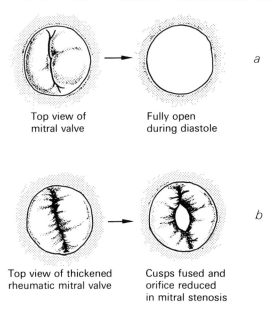

Top view of   Fully open
mitral valve   during diastole   *a*

Top view of thickened   Cusps fused and
rheumatic mitral valve   orifice reduced
                         in mitral stenosis   *b*

Fig. 6.2.   Mitral valve opening. (a) Normal. (b) Mitral stenosis.

aspirin. The ideal treatment is prevention, which starts with improving social conditions but includes treatment of the sore throat with penicillin. The incidence of rheumatic fever following a β-haemolytic sore throat is as low as 0.3 per cent and the bacteria are still totally sensitive to ordinary benzyl penicillin.

In the UK only about 50 per cent of patients who develop rheumatic heart disease have a history of rheumatic fever so many streptococcal infections may go undetected. Some patients will never have been told they had rheumatic fever but if questioned about 'growing pains' or a long absence from school will give a suggestive history. There is still a small but significant incidence of rheumatic fever in developed countries. Once a patient has had rheumatic fever he should be given penicillin either daily orally or monthly intramuscularly until he is about 25 years old.

Rheumatic fever primarily affects the mitral and aortic valves (? due to greater pressure on the left side of the heart) and the incidence of involvement is as follows:

Mitral valve   80 per cent
Aortic valve   30 per cent
Tricuspid valve ⎫
                 ⎬ less than 5 per cent
Pulmonary valve ⎭

2.   Congenital lesions (see chapter 7)

3.   Billowing mitral valve leaflet syndrome (Barlow's syndrome)

This valvular abnormality is very common and may affect as many as 10 per cent of females. One cusp of the valve may billow up into the left atrium with systole, causing a click or the cusp may slip back into the left atrium causing a click and systolic murmur. Occasionally the chordae of the cusp rupture altogether giving severe valvar incompetence (*Fig.* 6.3).

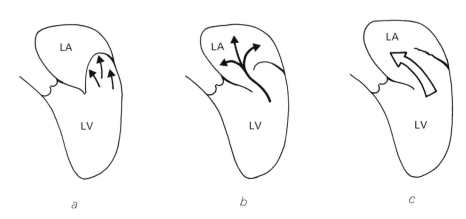

a   *b*   *c*

Fig. 6.3.   Stages in billowing mitral valve leaflet syndrome (Barlow's syndrome). (a) Billowing cusp of mitral valve. (b) Billowing cusp with mitral incompetence. (c) Prolapsed cusp of mitral valve.

In most cases of the billowing mitral valve leaflet syndrome the cause is not known although it does occur in some collagen diseases. Ruptured chordae may occur in infective endocarditis and after a myocardial infarction.

4.   Ischaemic heart disease

Because the papillary muscles tethering the mitral valve are part of the left ventricle they are often damaged by myocardial ischaemia or rendered less efficient. This usually causes mild mitral incompetence but rarely the muscles rupture and the leak may be severe and of acute onset. In heart failure the dilated ventricles result in stretched valve rings and, therefore, either mitral or tricuspid incompetence or sometimes both. This can often improve greatly with effective treatment of the failure.

5.   Other causes

Aortic incompetence: syphilis; dissecting aortic aneurysm; bacterial endocarditis; Marfan's syndrome.

Mitral incompetence: functional; bacterial endocarditis, connective tissue disease, e.g. rheumatoid arthritis.

● Clinical problems

Most valvular heart lesions can be diagnosed by symptoms and signs and the ECG, chest radiograph and echo will help to confirm the diagnosis. Cardiac catheterization may be necessary but is often performed in these cases to check for unsuspected coronary artery disease or to determine severity of valve lesions.

Occasionally the physical signs will lead one to suspect a valve lesion but in practice it can occasionally be subvalvular or even supravalvular. Pulmonary stenosis is often subvalvular (i.e. muscular hypertrophy obstructing the outflow tract of the right ventricle) and aortic stenosis can rarely be supravalvular or more commonly subvalvular.

Each valvular lesion is dealt with separately giving a brief outline of symptoms and the physical signs which specifically indicate that particular lesion. In practice many valvular lesions are mixed, i.e. stenosis and incompetence coexist and the physical signs become a mixture of the two lesions with possibly one or the other predominating. Likewise, more than one valve may be affected further altering the clinical picture.

Aortic stenosis

Symptoms

Once symptoms develop with aortic stenosis the outlook is limited and an operation is required. The symptoms of aortic stenosis can be called 'the 4 As' – Arrhythmias, Attacks of unconsciousness, Angina and Asthma (cardiac). A fixed cardiac output accounts for angina. Palpitations as well as attacks of unconsciousness may be directly related to abnormal rhythms. During exercise the peripheral resistance falls and the blood is preferentially diverted to skeletal muscles. Because the aortic valve is tight, the cardiac output fails to rise and the myocardium, as well as the brain, becomes ischaemic. As the stenosis tightens the left ventricle is under increasing strain until it fails and pulmonary oedema develops (cardiac asthma). The average survival time following the onset of symptoms is 2–3 years. Heart failure has the worst prognosis.

Signs

1.   The pulse. Characteristically the pulse is slow rising but this will only be apparent when the aortic stenosis is moderate to severe (see *Fig.* 3.5). In tight aortic stenosis the pulse pressure is reduced and therefore the pulse feels weak and of low volume.
2.   The blood pressure. As the stenosis increases the pulse pressure narrows. A typical blood pressure in severe aortic stenosis would be 105/90. It is not impossible, however, to get coexistent hypertension in patients with aortic stenosis but it is rare.
3.   Apex beat. The apex beat is described as sustained. It is easily felt, not usually displaced (hypertrophy occurs, not dilatation of the heart) and can characteristically be felt under the fingers for a long time. This is

because the ejection of blood through a small orifice requires a higher pressure and takes longer. The heart will dilate when failure ensues.

4.   The murmur and heart sounds. Aortic stenosis is heard in the 'aortic area'. This is not, however, where the aortic valve lies but where the turbulence occurs. The murmur is transmitted from here up into the neck. Because the pressure behind the aortic valve is enormous, the turbulence is violent and the murmur is harsh. At peak flow (mid systole) the turbulence is greatest and so the murmur is described as 'diamond shaped', 'crescendo-decrescendo' or simply 'ejection' type.

Mild aortic stenosis

The murmur is short. Aortic stenosis causes turbulence but if it is mild it only lasts a short time (*Fig.* 6.4).

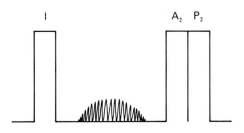

Fig. 6.4.   Mild aortic stenosis.

Moderate aortic stenosis

As the valve tightens the blood takes longer to get through and the murmur lengthens (*Fig.* 6.5).

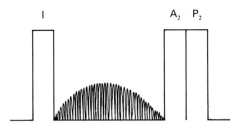

Fig. 6.5.   Moderate aortic stenosis.

Severe aortic stenosis

As the valve orifice becomes tiny, left ventricular ejection time exceeds right ventricular ejection time and A_2 occurs after P_2. This is called reverse splitting of

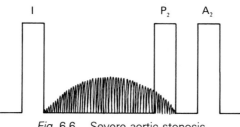

Fig. 6.6.   Severe aortic stenosis.

the second sound (*Fig.* 6.6). In practice the second sound may be very difficult to hear and differentiation from mitral regurgitation can be virtually impossible on auscultation.

A useful rule of thumb is that if the aortic stenotic murmur is harsh and the second sound is not heard, the lesion will be severe. If the second heart sound is clearly heard the lesion will be mild to moderate.

About 50 per cent of patients over the age of 50 years will have a flow murmur over the aortic outflow tract termed aortic sclerosis. One of the commonest causes of this is a stiffened aortic valve due to ageing. The murmur of aortic sclerosis is usually short with a clear second sound. The pulse pressure is usually wide as the sclerotic valve is associated with arteriosclerosis.

ECG
As aortic stenosis increases left ventricular hypertrophy and strain appear. On the ECG there is left ventricular hypertrophy (S wave in V_1 + R wave in V_5, V_6 = > 35 mm).

Chest radiography
Calcification may be seen in the area of the aortic valve and post-stenotic dilatation of the aorta may be found (*Fig.* 6.7). This is presumably an effect of the turbulence. The heart is not usually enlarged unless failure has developed.

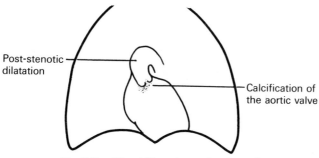

Fig. 6.7.   Chest X-ray in aortic stenosis.

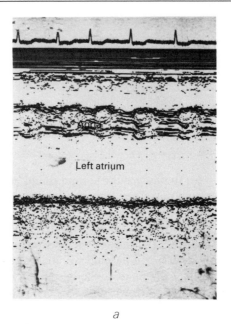

a

b

Fig. 6.8. Echocardiogram in aortic stenosis. Dense disorganized shadows are seen in the aorta and the valve is obscured. Left atrium is enlarged. (a) M-mode. (b) 2-D echocardiogram. LA = left atrium, LV = left ventricle, Ao = aorta, X = aortic valve calcification.

Echocardiography

Thickened left ventricular walls with a small left ventricular cavity are typical of severe aortic stenosis. This will be less obvious if the stenosis is milder. Dense shadows representing a thickened calcified valve may be seen as echoes traversing the aortic root (*Fig.* 6.8). Two-dimensional echocardiographs can now well demonstrate the restricted movement of the valve leaflets and give a very accurate measurement of the severity of the stenosis.

Cardiac catheter

Pressure in the left ventricle rises higher than in the aorta in an effort to eject the left ventricular contents in the time allocated (*Fig.* 6.9). The difference in pressure is called the aortic valve gradient which is regarded as severe if it is 70 mmHg or more. Surgery is usually indicated for gradients in excess of 50 mmHg but the range 50–70 mmHg is more of a grey area in terms of benefit.

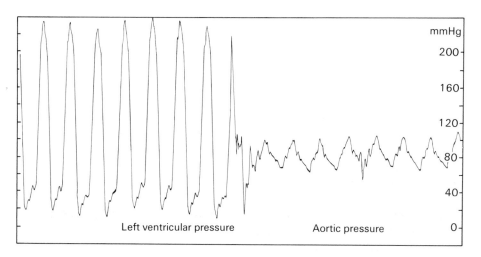

Fig. 6.9.   Recording of pressure as catheter is pulled back from left ventricle to aorta in aortic stenosis.

Aortic incompetence

Symptoms

Every cardiac symptom occurs with aortic incompetence and unlike aortic stenosis their appearance does not represent impending disaster. Patients with aortic incompetence can go on for many years without deterioration. Judging the time of surgical intervention is still controversial but depends quite a lot on the patient's symptoms.

Signs

A patient with aortic incompetence is a pleasure to examine because of the plethora of physical signs.

1. Collapsing pulse. The pulse pressure in aortic incompetence is wide because a high proportion of the ejected blood falls back into the left ventricle and the diastolic pressure falls. The definition of a collapsing pulse is if pulse pressure exceeds the diastolic pressure. The pulse feels as though it is rapidly disappearing and is thus called 'collapsing' (see *Fig.* 3.5).

2. Waterhammer pulse. If the arm is held above the level of the heart the radial pulse feels tapping in nature because the diastolic fall is accentuated. It is called a waterhammer pulse after a Victorian toy. This was a glass rod half filled with a liquid and half filled with a vacuum. As the glass rod was turned vertically, the fluid hit the end of the glass with a gentle tap. This is likened to the pulse.

3. Corrigan's sign. Corrigan, an Irish physician, remarked on the striking feature of pulsating carotid arteries in severe aortic incompetence.

4. Quinke's sign or nailbed pulsation. Light pressure on the tip of the nails demonstrates capillary pulsation in patients with moderate to severe aortic incompetence.

5. De Musset's sign. De Musset, a French beggar, had such severe aortic incompetence that every time his carotid vessels filled with blood his head moved up. He, therefore, nodded in time with his pulse and this is known as his sign. It is very rare.

6. Dancing retinal arteries. On retinoscopy, the retinal vessels can be seen to pulsate.

7. Pistol shot femorals. Gentle auscultation over the femoral arteries reveals a sudden crack in time with systole. This is due to the sudden rapid expansion of the arteries.

8. Durosiez's sign. A systolic bruit is heard over the femoral arteries if light pressure is produced using the leading edge of the stethoscope (*Fig.* 6.10).

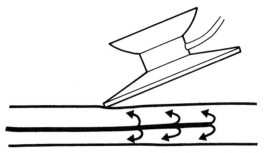

Fig. 6.10.   Technique for eliciting Durosiez's sign.

A diastolic bruit is heard over the femoral artery when light pressure is produced by the distal edge of the stethoscope. This is because blood is flowing back to the heart in diastole and the pressure causes turbulence under the stethoscope (*Fig.* 6.11). This is a useful physical sign because it suggests severe aortic incompetence.

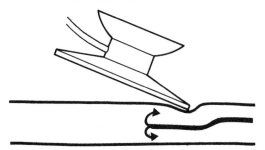

Fig. 6.11. Audible turbulence in aortic incompetence when the stethoscope is in reverse position to Fig. 6.10.

9. Blood pressure. A wide pulse pressure is present because so much blood falls back into the left ventricle during diastole. The diastolic pressure may become virtually 0 in severe cases of aortic incompetence.
10. Apex beat. The left ventricle dilates so that it can eject a larger stroke volume. If the regurgitant volume is 50 per cent it will have to eject twice the normal volume to maintain a normal cardiac output. Because there is no pressure overload in aortic incompetence there is only moderate ventricular hypertrophy.
11. The murmur. Blood passes back into the left ventricle through an incompetent valve and the diastolic pressure rapidly falls. The murmur is, therefore, decrescendo and soft. It is best heard in the area of turbulence, i.e. the 3rd and 4th left intercostal spaces. An ejection systolic murmur may also be heard which does not necessarily mean there is accompanying *aortic* stenosis. It is due to the large volume of blood being ejected over the aortic valve. When aortic incompetence is trivial the murmur is short (*Fig.* 6.12).

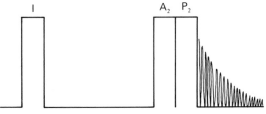

Fig. 6.12. Mild aortic incompetence.

As the degree of incompetence increases blood flows into the ventricle for an increasing time (*Fig.* 6.13). When left ventricular failure sets in the left ventricular end diastolic pressure rises and curtails the regurgitation. The murmur begins to shorten again. This represents severe aortic incompetence.

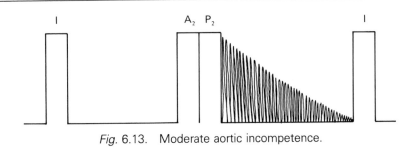

Fig. 6.13.   Moderate aortic incompetence.

ECG
A diastolic overload pattern is seen. There is left ventricular hypertrophy with tall T waves in leads V_5 and V_6.

Chest radiograph
Calcification may be visible in the area of the aortic valve but the most obvious sign is a large heart and dilated aorta.

Echocardiography
A large dilated vigorous left ventricular cavity is present until the late stages when, if an operation is not performed, the muscle becomes weak and left ventricular contraction poor. The incompetent aortic valve is not directly visualized. An end systolic volume of greater than 5.5 cm may be an indication for operation. Doppler ultrasound can quantify the leak.

Cardiac catheter
When dye is rapidly injected into the aorta just above the aortic valve it will regurgitate into the left ventricle if aortic incompetence is present. The amount of dye falling back into the left ventricle is an indication of the severity of aortic incompetence (*Fig.* 6.14).

Mitral stenosis

Symptoms
Almost every cardiac symptom occurs in mitral stenosis. In addition, because of the presence of pulmonary hypertension, bronchitis is common, and fatigue is particularly prominent. Like aortic incompetence, surgical intervention is mainly based on symptoms.

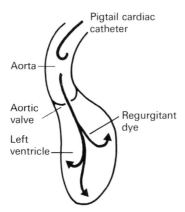

Fig. 6.14.   Angiography in aortic incompetence.

Patients with mitral stenosis are very prone to develop atrial fibrillation. This may cause a sudden deterioration in symptoms and is frequently associated with systemic embolism if not treated with anticoagulation. Atrial fibrillation starts relatively early (average age 28 years) presumably due to left atrial dilatation. Thrombus develops in the large atrium and emboli pass into the circulation at the rate of 4 per cent per annum in patients not on anticoagulants.

Signs
1.   Mitral facies. A plethoric colour over the malar area is a classic sign in mitral valve disease although it tends to occur late. It is called a 'malar flush'.
2.   'Tapping' apex beat. In mitral stenosis the left ventricle is small and often barely felt and when it is it feels like a tap. A loud first heart sound may be palpable also.
3.   Right ventricular heave. Mitral stenosis leads to a high left atrial pressure and subsequently to both high pulmonary venous and pulmonary arterial pressures. Right ventricular hypertrophy results and gives a ventricular heave.
4.   Heart sounds and murmurs. A loud first sound is heard in mitral stenosis because of the sudden cessation of diastolic flow and closure of the mitral valve. The cusps remain fully open under the high left atrial pressure until the sudden rise in left ventricular pressure at the start of systole. Once the cusps become rigid, and allow some regurgitation, this sign disappears. A loud pulmonary second sound indicates the presence of pulmonary hypertension.

The murmur of mitral stenosis is a low pitched, rumbling mid-diastolic murmur, localized to the apex and heard best with the patient lying on the left side. This murmur is caused by turbulence through the stenosed

valve, and does not radiate. When the cusps spring open due to the high
left atrial pressure a sound is made which is called the opening snap (*Fig.
6.15*). The closer the opening snap is to the second sound then the tighter
the mitral valve stenosis. When the valve becomes thick and calcified no
such opening is possible and the opening snap disappears.

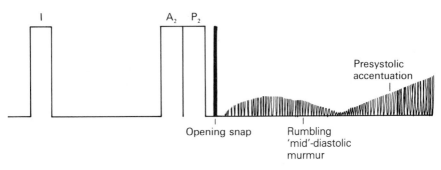

Fig. 6.15.   Mitral stenosis.

The murmur of mitral stenosis increases just before the second sound (the
presystolic murmur accentuation) and is said to be due to atrial contraction. This
is only partially true although the murmur is commonly absent in atrial
fibrillation. Its main cause is the pliability of the mitral cusps and, therefore, it
can still be heard in patients who are fibrillating.

There are two important points when assessing mitral stenosis:

1.   Severity of lesion. As left atrial pressure rises due to greater stenosis, the
murmur starts closer to the second sound.
2.   Pliability of the valve. As the valve becomes stiff and calcified, a mitral
valvotomy or valvuloplasty becomes less practicable. A pliable valve
gives a loud first heart sound, crisp opening snap and an easily heard
presystolic murmur.

ECG

Left atrial enlargement gives P mitrale and as the left atrial pressure rises right
ventricular hypertrophy may be seen. Many patients develop atrial fibrillation
and are given digoxin, the effect of which can often be seen on the ECG.

Chest radiography

In pure mitral stenosis the heart is compact on radiography but with a large left
atrium. This is seen as a double shadow on the right border of the heart, a
prominence on the left border and a splaying of the carina (see *Fig.* 4.12).

As pulmonary hypertension develops the pulmonary arteries will enlarge
and the right ventricle may become enormous. Pulmonary oedema may develop

in tight mitral stenosis. Calcification of the mitral valve is seen late in the disease.

Echocardiography

Mitral stenosis can be seen directly on the echo. Instead of the normal 'M'-shaped configuration of the valve (*Fig.* 6.16) it opens less, closes more slowly and shows no peaks while the posterior cusp moves anteriorly as the valve

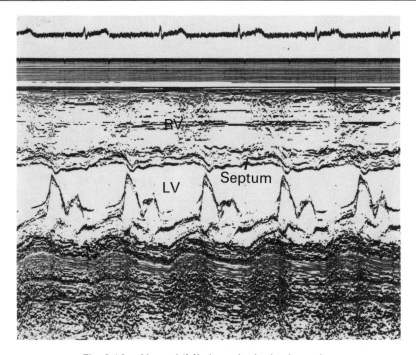

Fig. 6.16.   Normal 'M'-shaped mitral valve echo.

opens (*Fig.* 6.17). The reduction in closing rate correlates with the severity of the mitral stenosis. 2-D echocardiography demonstrates the reduced valve area and ballooning of the valve (*Fig.* 6.18).

Cardiac catheter

Simultaneous left atrial and left ventricular tracings show a gradient during diastole (*Fig.* 6.19).

Mitral incompetence

The commonest causes of mitral incompetence (rheumatic fever and billowing mitral leaflet syndrome) produce different murmurs but the symptoms and signs are essentially similar.

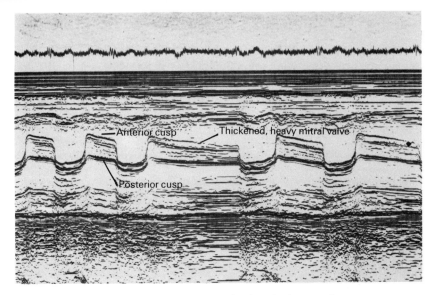

Fig. 6.17.   Mitral valve echo in mitral stenosis.

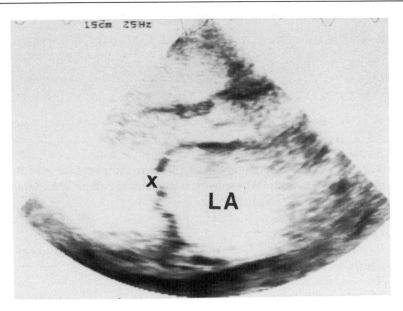

Fig. 6.18.   Ballooning mitral valve (x) and enlarged left atrium (LA) seen on 2-D echocardiogram in mitral stenosis.

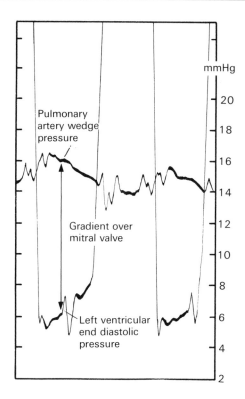

Fig. 6.19.   Simultaneous pressures recorded from either side of the mitral valve (PAW = LA) show a pressure gradient over the valve = mitral stenosis.

Symptoms

Any cardiac symptom may develop with mitral incompetence. Palpitations are frequent because the heart is often very large and easily felt against the chest wall. Palpitations occur more commonly with the billowing mitral leaflet syndrome and although these can represent significant arrhythmias death is extremely uncommon. Left-sided chest pain of unknown cause, perhaps cardiac neurosis, occurs with the billowing mitral leaflet, particularly in young women. Whatever the cause of mitral incompetence, symptoms increase as the lesion becomes more severe and surgical intervention is according to these.

Signs

1.   Mitral facies, see mitral stenosis.
2.   Diffuse heaving apex beat. The left ventricle becomes dilated and vigorous as the stroke volume increases. As the incompetence becomes severe half the stroke volume may go into the left atrium and a mini collapsing pulse may be felt.

3. Left atrial 'kick'. A second 'kick' felt over the sternum immediately following the right ventricular heave represents a left atrial 'kick'. It is due to the rapid filling from the left ventricle and because the left atrium cannot expand posteriorly (the vertebral column prevents it) the sternum is pushed forward slightly. This sign only appears in severe mitral incompetence.

4. Right ventricular heave. High right ventricular pressure due to pulmonary hypertension is common in mitral incompetence.

5. Heart sounds and murmurs – mitral incompetence. The first heart sound is usually soft because the cusps do not approximate precisely, and there is no sudden cessation of blood flow.

The murmur. From the start of systole blood pours into the left atrium and continues until systole ends. The murmur is therefore pansystolic. Although there is great pressure in the left ventricle the murmur is soft because the orifice (i.e. the valvular incompetence) is large. The murmur is heard best over the mitral region but is transmitted widely, particularly to the axilla, perhaps because the left atrium acts as a reflecting bowl. When the incompetence is severe blood pours into the left atrium during systole and rushes back in diastole giving a third heart sound. If the cusps are distorted (i.e. in rheumatic heart disease) a short diastolic murmur may also be heard (*Fig.* 6.20).

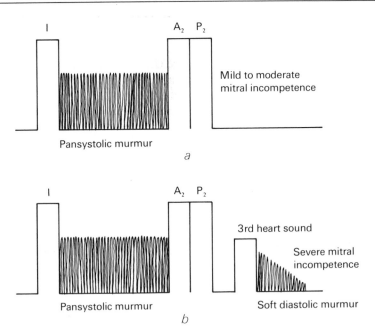

Fig. 6.20. (a) Mild to moderate mitral incompetence. (b) Severe mitral incompetence.

6. The murmur – billowing mitral leaflet syndrome. This syndrome, also called the 'click murmur' syndrome, may present with a click alone (probably a normal variant) which causes no haemodynamic problems to the heart or a click and murmur with varying degrees of valvular incompetence. The click is heard in the same area as rheumatic mitral incompetence (*Fig.* 6.21).

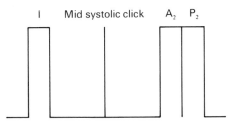

Fig. 6.21. Typical timing of the systolic click in the billowing mitral leaflet syndrome.

When the syndrome becomes more severe the billowing cusp prolapses into the left atrium and allows mitral incompetence. The click is then followed by a murmur (*Fig.* 6.22). The murmur has a characteristic 'whoop' sometimes likened to a cooing dove.

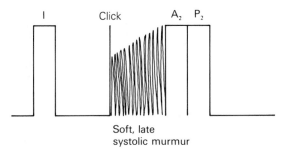

Soft, late
systolic murmur

Fig. 6.22. Sounds and murmur in the billowing mitral leaflet syndrome when the valve is also leaking.

ECG

Left ventricular hypertrophy is seen with a diastolic overload pattern (see Aortic incompetence). P mitrale may be seen. In the billowing mitral valve leaflet syndrome non-specific T wave changes may occur, particularly in the inferior leads.

Chest radiography

There is left ventricular enlargement with an increased cardiothoracic ratio and a double right heart border may be seen suggestive of left atrial enlargement. The pulmonary arteries may enlarge and pulmonary oedema may be seen. Calcification of the mitral valve is seen late in the disease.

Echocardiography

Mitral incompetence can be detected and quantified by Doppler echocardiography. 2-D echocardiograms show the left ventricle to be enlarged and to move vigorously. The left atrium will become large. The billowing mitral leaflet is directly visualized during systole by the posterior motion of one cusp (*Fig.* 6.23).

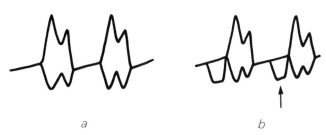

a   *b*

Fig. 6.23.   Diagram of echo. (a) Showing normal M shape. (b) Prolapsing mitral valve leaflet (arrowed).

Cardiac catheter

During a left ventriculogram dye will be seen to enter the left atrium during systole. The quantity which goes into the left atrium can be assessed visually and the severity of the incompetence calculated.

Tricuspid stenosis

Symptoms

This rare valve lesion causes right-sided heart problems – liver congestion and peripheral oedema in particular. The patient may notice right hypochondrial pain, a full feeling in the abdomen after meals, ankle swelling and abdominal swelling (ascites).

Signs

1.   Raised jugular venous pressure. This is very high and the ear lobes may be seen 'waggling'.
2.   Enlarged tender liver. This may be 4 or 5 cm below the costal margin and feels very uncomfortable.
3.   Ankle or sacral oedema.
4.   The murmur. The murmur is similar to that of mitral stenosis but is heard in the tricuspid area.

ECG
Right atrial enlargement (P pulmonale) may be seen.

Chest radiography
The heart size may be normal but the right atrial enlargement may cause some increase in cardiothoracic ratio. Tricuspid stenosis rarely occurs alone and usually there is evidence of other valve involvement.

Echocardiography
The tricuspid valve is changed to the same shape as in mitral stenosis.

Cardiac catheter
Simultaneous right atrial and right ventricular pressure will reveal a valvular gradient.

Tricuspid incompetence
Tricuspid incompetence is usually functional, i.e. due to a dilated valve ring secondary to right ventricular distension in heart failure. It is quite a common occurrence but may be reversible. Treatment of heart failure will often result in disappearance of the signs.

Symptoms
As for tricuspid stenosis but if tricuspid incompetence is severe a pulsation in the neck may be felt from the constant venous waves in the jugular veins.

Signs
1.   Jugular venous pressure. The jugular venous pressure will be raised and will also show large 'v' waves.
2.   Enlarged, tender, pulsatile liver. The pulsation results from the 'v' wave which is readily transmitted back to the liver.
3.   Ankle or sacral oedema.
4.   Murmur. Similar to that of mitral incompetence but the intensity of the murmur varies with respiration. As the patient breathes in more blood comes to the right side of the heart and the incompetence is apparently greater. The murmur, therefore, increases with inspiration and decreases with expiration. It is best heard over the lower end of the sternum.

ECG
Right ventricular and right atrial enlargement will be seen.

Chest radiography
The heart is usually very large as the right ventricle and right atrium distend.

Echocardiography
A large right ventricle will be seen and Doppler ultrasound will detect the leak.

Cardiac catheter

A large 'v' wave may be recorded from the right atrium.

● Treatment of valvular heart disease

There is no direct medical treatment of the valve itself except to limit rheumatic fever if it is present and to prevent its recurrence. Direct treatment of the valve is surgical or by interventional cardiac catheter techniques. Medical treatment is aimed at the complications of the valvular problem.

1. Heart failure

Treatment of acute or chronic congestive cardiac failure is made along conventional lines, i.e. digoxin, diuretics, etc. (see chapter 10).

2. Arrhythmias

Any arrhythmia must be treated if it is life threatening or causing cardiac failure. Mitral valve disease frequently causes atrial fibrillation, which can be treated with digoxin or other anti-arrhythmics. A common complication of mitral valve disease and atrial fibrillation is a systemic embolus and most patients with mitral valve disease, especially stenosis, are anticoagulated.

3. Pulmonary hypertension

Mitral or aortic valve disease may result in pulmonary hypertension and the development of this is one factor precipitating valve replacement. Medical therapy does not directly influence pulmonary hypertension but treatment of heart failure may reduce it somewhat.

4. Infective endocarditis

Antibiotic treatment for this is discussed elsewhere and because infective endocarditis still carries a high mortality, prevention is a very important aspect.

● Surgical treatment of valvular heart disease

1. Valvotomy

This is an uncommon operation now and is almost limited to the mitral valve. A finger or Tubbs dilator opens up the valve along the fissure line and it can be a very successful operation. Once the valve is thickened and calcified the procedure is more hazardous so that the operation is limited to tight pliable mitral stenosis. Aortic valvotomies are carried out in children and sometimes in young adults.

2.   Valve reconstruction

Direct repair of a valve or reduction of the size of the valve ring (called annuloplasty) is only possible if the valve itself is almost normal. Reattachment of ruptured chordae tendinae and reversal of mitral incompetence by reduction of the ring size are operations with a reasonable amount of success.

3.   Valve replacement

This is easily the commonest valve operation. A prosthetic valve replaces the natural valve which is removed in its entirety. It is now an operation which carries a low mortality. Valves may be homografts (using a valve constructed from the patient's own tissue, e.g. fascia lata), xenograft (e.g. pig heart valves) or synthetic valves (see *Fig.* 6.24).

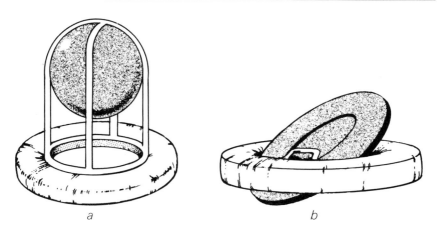

a   *b*

Fig. 6.24.   (a) Starr–Edwards prosthesis. (b) Björk–Shiley prosthesis.

The timing of a valve replacement depends predominantly on symptoms and is particular for the individual. Signs of strain on the ECG or excessive enlargement of the heart on chest radiography may also hasten surgery. Generally speaking (except for aortic stenosis) the patient with valvular heart disease who cannot get up one flight of stairs without stopping needs an operation.

4.   Valvuloplasty

In recent years balloon dilatation of stenosed valves has become possible. The balloon is inserted using standard cardiac catheter techniques and when astride the relevant valve is inflated thus effectively performing a valvotomy. It is the treatment of choice for congenital pulmonary stenosis and has some part to play in mitral or aortic stenosis.

Replacement heart valves

	Advantages	*Disadvantages*
1. Homograft valve	Anticoagulants not needed	Stenosis and scar after a few years
2. Xenograft valve (pig valve)	Good flow ? Anticoagulants not needed	May become stiff or fibrosed
3. Synthetic valve (a) Starr–Edwards (ball and cage) (titanium)	Robust	Needs anticoagulation Causes haemolysis Considerable obstruction to flow
(b) Björk–Shiley (tilting disc)	Robust Fairly good flow	Needs anticoagulation
(c) St Jude (double opening disc – carbon pyrolyte)	Robust Excellent flow	Needs anticoagulation

7

Congenital heart disease

Congenital heart disease is becoming increasingly relevant to the daily practice of cardiology because many of these neonates or children can now be palliated or corrected and so are going on to adult life where an ever-growing number of them are attending adult clinics.

About 8 per 1000 live births are of children with congenital heart disease. It is highly likely that many more potential cases of congenital heart disease are spontaneously aborted by the mother. If parents have one affected child their chances of having another similarly affected are increased to about 25 per 1000 live births. This, in the absence of an obvious cause for the heart problem, is not a substantially greater risk than that of the general population and the parents can be reassured to a large extent.

It is probably better to think of neonatal congenital heart disease separately from heart problems or murmurs detected later in life. The incidence of the various disorders is quite different at this age.

● **Neonatal congenital heart disease**

These patients present with either heart failure or cyanosis. Heart failure in neonates is more subtle than in adults and a search should be made for hepatomegaly, poor pulses, tachycardia, tachypnoea, signs of fluid in the lungs and excessive weight gain. Clearly good charting of the baby's pulse, respiration and weight by the nurses is vital for detecting trends. The doctor's most useful contribution is to detect hepatomegaly and to listen to the lung fields. The latter is often the least helpful.

Cyanosis is very common in babies. Even the most healthy of children are 'blue at the edges' when cold. However, there is a generalized duskiness to truly centrally cyanosed infants which is fairly characteristic when one is used to looking for it. Cyanosis may be respiratory in nature and not due to heart disease. On the other hand, babies with hypoxia often reopen their ductus arteriosus and hence may develop heart failure from this.

Examination

1. *Inspection*
Examination of these young children should include close inspection for signs such as costal indrawing and tachypnoea. Cyanosis will be spotted and sometimes the liver can be seen showing through the abdominal wall.

2. *Pulses*
All the peripheral pulses should be felt. In patent ductus arteriosus there is a wide pulse pressure and the pulses are 'bouncy' or collapsing. This is especially easy to feel in the femoral pulses and is a most useful sign. 'Bouncy' pulses should equal a patent ductus until otherwise proven as other causes of this sign such as truncus arteriosus or aortic incompetence are relatively rare. Poor pulses in the legs may be felt in coarctation of the aorta. In this case the pulses, at least in the right arm, will be easily felt.

3. *Blood pressure*
Blood pressure is difficult to take in neonates and is often inaccurate.

4. *Auscultation*
The heart sounds should be listened to and in particular it should be determined whether the second sound is split or not. Murmurs heard in neonates are usually systolic and because of the rapid heart rate it is difficult to sort out ejection from pansystolic murmurs. The most important thing about a murmur in a neonate is to detect its presence. Diastolic murmurs are rare and even the patent ductus murmur tends not to be the continuous machinery murmur heard so characteristically in older children, but simply to be an ejection systolic murmur even in the largest ducts. In general, murmurs heard within the first 24–48 hours of life are due to obstructive lesions such as aortic stenosis and those first heard later are more likely to be due to defects in the ventricular (or less often) atrial septa. Early in life the right- and left-sided pressures are more or less equal and so there is little flow over shunts. Only when the pulmonary vascular resistance drops does shunt flow increase and the murmur appear. Parents are often amazed that their child's ventricular septal defect has been missed by the examining paediatrician in hospital and only noticed sometime later by their own doctor.

5. *ECG*
The ECG should always be done but there is rather a wide range of normality in its criteria and it is not a particularly sensitive index.

6. *Chest radiograph*

The chest radiograph is helpful but normal heart size may be up to 60 per cent of thoracic width in neonates. There are characteristic shapes such as the boot shape of Fallot's tetralogy. The vascularity of the lung fields should be checked. In assessing the vascularity of lung fields the size of the small bronchi should be the same as the equivalent pulmonary arteries. Lung markings should be difficult to detect beyond the outer third of the lung fields. If markings are seen at the periphery of the lungs then it is likely that there is increased blood flow to the lungs.

7. *Echocardiography*

M-mode echocardiography revolutionized the diagnosis of neonatal congenital heart disease. All the valves and all the chambers should be able to be demonstrated together with the great vessels. If they are not seen then they are likely not to be there. There are not the same problems with echocardiography in children as can be the case with adults. Children are much easier to examine in this way. Two-dimensional echocardiography and, more recently, Doppler ultrasound have further improved diagnosis and lesions such as ventricular and atrial septal defects can be visualized and coarctations of the aorta delineated. In some cases echoes have completely eliminated the need for cardiac catheterization.

Specific lesions causing heart failure

Hypoplastic left heart is as the name suggests. It is the commonest neonatal lesion presenting with heart failure. Nothing can be done about this condition apart from treating the failure. Other lesions causing heart failure are coarctation of the aorta, aortic stenosis of the congenital kind where the valves are myxomatous and hardly formed, truncus arteriosus, double outlet right ventricle and severe endocardial cushion defects. Several lesions may occur together and unless one is aware of this possibility it is easily overlooked. It is not all that uncommon to find neonates with an atrial septal defect, ventricular septal defect and patent ductus arteriosus. Together these can add up to a collosal shunt with severe heart failure.

Specific lesions causing cyanosis

Transposition of the great arteries is the commonest cause of neonatal congenital cyanotic heart disease. These children are often dependent on their ductus arteriosus allowing communication between the pulmonary and systemic blood circulations. Often the cyanosis comes and goes as the ductus attempts to close and then the ensuing hypoxia reopens it. Pulmonary atresia (absent pulmonary valve) with or without a ventricular septal defect, total anomalous pulmonary venous return and tricuspid atresia are other causes of neonatal cyanosis.

Notice that this list of conditions is altogether different from that seen in older children and until recently most of these lesions were rapidly fatal.

Nowadays the majority are amenable to surgery so some knowledge of these defects will be required by cardiologists and physicians, and even family doctors.

● **Congenital heart disease in older children**
Conventionally this is divided into cyanotic and acyanotic congenital heart disease. Since acyanotic forms are much commoner they will be described first.

Acyanotic congenital heart disease

Ventricular septal defect (VSD)
This is the commonest form of congenital heart disease and is about 25 per cent of the total. There is a defect in the ventricular septum which usually lies high up in the membranous part although less frequently the defect is found in the muscular part. Occasionally there are multiple defects (*Fig. 7.1*).

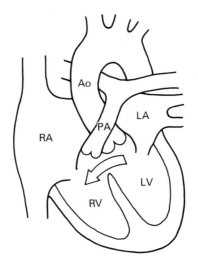

Fig. 7.1. Ventricular septal defect.

Because left ventricular pressure is higher than right ventricular pressure blood flows from left to right across the defect. Thirty to 50 per cent of ventricular septal defects will close spontaneously, the great majority of them doing so in the first year of life. Even large defects with torrential flow through them can close and it is not possible on the basis of shunt size to say which defect will close spontaneously and which will not. As the child grows the heart gets larger around the defect so that the defect, which may not change in size, becomes relatively smaller.

Heart failure

Large ventricular septal defects can cause heart failure at any time. In patients with VSDs the pulmonary artery pressure tends to stay high, as it is in the fetus, for 1 or 2 months following birth. It then falls and with this fall the flow of blood through the VSD can increase substantially so that heart failure is common at this time. Medical therapy is vigorous in order to try and tide the child over this period in the hope that the defect will become smaller or disappear. Occasionally it does not and the VSD has to be closed surgically. In children under 6 months of age this operation has a higher risk compared with that in older children and for this reason many surgeons prefer palliative surgery where a band is placed around the pulmonary artery to raise the right ventricular pressure and stop the torrential flow of blood to the lungs. Later on the band is removed and the VSD repaired.

ECG and chest radiograph

Most children are asymptomatic and are followed-up frequently to detect the onset of pulmonary hypertension. The ECG is relatively sensitive in this regard, and in lead V_1 in particular, if the T wave becomes flat or upright the pulmonary artery pressure ought to be checked and the defect closed if pulmonary hypertension is developing; similarly with cardiomegaly on the chest radiograph. The lung fields are, of course, plethoric.

Heart sounds and murmurs

Clinically the children usually appear normal. The heart may be enlarged but the children are not usually in overt failure. The heart sounds are usually normal although where pulmonary hypertension is developing P_2 may be loud. There is a pansystolic murmur best heard at the left sternal edge in the 3rd and 4th interspace. It may radiate elsewhere. Clinically it is most useful to listen for an apical mid diastolic murmur (more like a rumble) (*Fig.* 7.2). This is due to the increased blood flow over the mitral valve and usually means that blood flow to the lungs is at least twice that of the systemic circulation. This is an important point becuase shunts of more than 2:1 should usually be closed surgically.

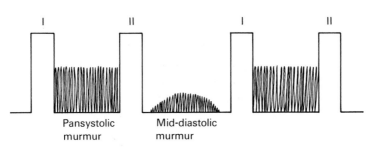

Fig. 7.2.   Heart sounds and murmurs of significant ventricular septal defect.

Surgery

The timing of surgery is under some dispute. It is best to avoid it if at all possible in the first year in the hope that the defect will close. If not, pulmonary hypertension starts to develop in the second year and it is usual to close shunts of more than 2:1 at this time. In shunts of less than 2:1 the patient is not likely to develop pulmonary hypertension and the albeit slight risk from surgery is greater than the risk of leaving the VSD unclosed.

Shunts requiring surgical closure may have:

1. Mitral flow murmur
2. Cardiomegaly clinically and radiologically with plethoric lung fields
3. Right or biventricular hypertrophy on the ECG

Echocardiography

The VSD may be identified by two-dimensional echocardiography in younger patients and circumstantial evidence (right ventricular volume overload) seen in others. Doppler echocardiography may detect the abnormal flow through the defect and into the right ventricle.

Untreated VSDs in the past used to develop pulmonary hypertension with eventual shunting from the right side of the heart to the left and cyanosis (Eisenmenger's syndrome). They died in the third to fourth decade of life.

Atrial septal defect (ASD) (*Fig. 7.3*)

There are basically two major types of atrial septal defect (ASD): the ostium secundum defect which tends to be a distinct embryological entity and the ostium primum defect which is part of the spectrum of lesions associated with endocardial cushion defects. The distinction is important because ostium secundum defects tend to be the sole abnormality while with ostium primum

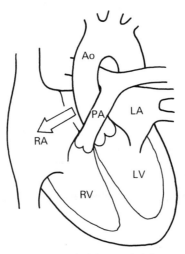

Fig. 7.3.   Atrial septal defect.

defects there may be associated abnormalities of the mitral valve (cleft mitral valve which may sometimes be incompetent), tricuspid valve and interventricular septum. Clinically they are hard to differentiate but fortunately they give quite different patterns on the ECG and echocardiogram. It is the findings with these two non-invasive investigations that would require a cardiac catheterization to be performed on an ostium primum defect whereas with an ostium secundum defect you might well send the child straight for surgical correction.

Clinical presentation

Usually these patients are symptom-free, the abnormality being detected on routine examination. The murmurs of this lesion are easily overlooked but if the second sound is sought and fixed or wide splitting is listened for then this is a great help. There is usually an ejection systolic murmur at the pulmonary area which is due solely to the increased flow over this valve. The blood traversing the actual ASD itself does not make any sound. In shunts of more than 2:1 pulmonary to systemic blood flow there is often a tricuspid flow murmur (*Fig. 7.4*). This is a diastolic rumble and suggests a significant left to right flow of blood.

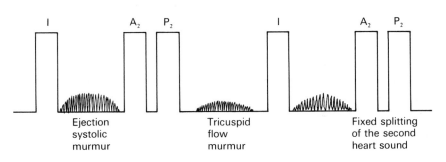

Fig. 7.4.   Heart sounds and murmurs of significant atrial septal defect.

In patients with ostium primum defects there may be pansystolic murmurs of mitral reflux or of a ventricular septal defect, or both. Ostium secundum atrial septal defects seldom cause heart failure in early life. For reasons that are not clear pulmonary hypertension in secundum defects develops later, usually during the second decade. It is usually not necessary, therefore, to keep such a close eye on these patients in early life as it is with ventricular septal defects.

Pulmonary hypertension develops earlier with ostium primum or partial endocardial cushion defects and these patients have to be investigated and treated earlier than those with secundum defects.

Chest radiograph

In both types of ASD the heart on radiography tends to be full or enlarged, the lung fields are plethoric with prominent main pulmonary arteries. The aorta is small as is the left ventricle and the absence of an obvious aorta together with large pulmonary arteries on the chest radiograph is virtually diagnostic.

ECG

The ECG is most helpful. There is usually at least partial right bundle branch block seen in lead V_1. Ostium primum defects have left axis deviation on the ECG and often a prolonged PR interval. Ostium secundum defects have a right axis and usually a normal PR interval.

Echocardiography

The echocardiogram in secundum defects suggests right ventricular volume overload. This is also seen with primum defects but in addition the mitral valve is usually abnormally highly placed and its anterior leaflet may be seen to pass through the ventricular septum. With two-dimensional echocardiography the defect may be identified and located but only clearly up to about the age of 4 years.

Cardiac catheterization

Left ventricular angiography shows the typical 'goose neck' appearance which is caused by the abnormally high mitral valve in primum defects. In secundum ASDs the left ventricle is normal in shape.

Large ASDs are closed surgically. Spontaneous closure does not occur and if left untreated pulmonary hypertension develops in the teenager and death follows in the fourth or fifth decade.

Patent ductus arteriosus (PDA)

The ductus arteriosus is very important physiologically *in utero* carrying, as it does, oxygenated blood from the placenta via the right ventricle over into the systemic side of the circulation (*Fig.* 7.5). It becomes redundant at birth when the placental circulation is lost and the lungs expand. Usually it closes

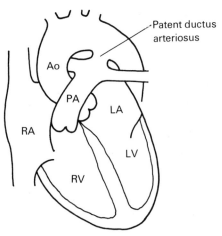

Fig. 7.5.   Patent ductus arteriosus.

functionally within 24 hours of birth and structurally within 1 or 2 weeks. This functional closure in response to a high blood PO_2 then becomes an anatomical closure and permanent. However, early in life the ductus can reopen in response to hypoxia and this is frequently seen in premature infants who have respiratory problems. It then becomes very difficult to judge how much the ductus is contributing to the general clinical picture. If small and seemingly insignificant the ductus should be left alone in the hope that it will close. It may be large enough to cause heart failure in which case indomethacin orally or intravenously may work or else the duct should be ligated surgically, a very low risk procedure. Such neonates have 'bouncy' or collapsing pulses, an ejection murmur in the pulmonary area that tends to come and go, possibly plethoric lung fields and an enlarged left atrium on the echocardiogram.

Two-dimensional echocardiographs may identify the lesion while Doppler demonstrates turbulence and abnormal flow in the pulmonary artery.

The more classic description of patent ductus arteriosus is seen in the older child. Usually they have developed normally and are symptom-free but have large volume pulses. The murmur is usually discovered on routine examination and typically is a systolic ejection type of murmur with a rough diastolic murmur in the pulmonary area. It sounds very much like a ship's engine-room, hence the term 'machinery murmur'. Even small ducts are closed surgically because of the high risk of bacterial endocarditis. The chest radiograph and ECGs are often normal although if the duct is large the heart will be enlarged and the lung fields plethoric on radiography. In such cases there will be right ventricular hypertrophy on the ECG.

Such patients are often sent direct to surgery although every now and again an irate surgeon will have an aortopulmonary window to close instead of a ductus. It is not worth cardiac catheters in all patients to find the odd window pre-operatively and in any event this is much less of a problem with 2-D echocardiography.

Untreated pulmonary hypertension used to develop, with larger shunts, around the second decade with death in the fourth or fifth decade.

Classically at cardiac catheterization the catheter passes down the ductus and into the descending aorta. Often this happens when investigating other cardiac anomalies and the route that the catheter takes comes as something of a surprise, a patent ductus being present in addition. Some patent ductuses in older children and young adults have been closed by means of devices on the end of cardiac catheters. These are rather umbrella like and when opened at the mouth of the ductus close it.

Aortic stenosis

This may present in the neonatal period with severe obstruction to the left ventricular outflow. The valve is usually grossly abnormal and deformed and because of this the operative mortality is very high at around 50 per cent. The echocardiogram is very helpful in making the diagnosis in which case the valve cannot be identified.

Clinical presentation

Much more common is aortic stenosis detected on routine examination later in life when a murmur is heard. The valve often has only two cusps (bicuspid aortic valve) instead of the usual three (*Fig.* 7.6). Bicuspid aortic valves are very common in the population (estimated 1–5 per cent) but aortic stenosis is rare by comparison. The child is usually normal and asymptomatic although some present with syncope on exertion. Unlike in adults angina and heart failure (after the neonatal period) are uncommon. On examination there may be a systolic thrill radiating to the neck and the apex beat may feel sustained.

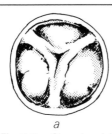 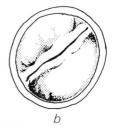

a   *b*

Fig. 7.6.   Showing (a) normal aortic valve; (b) bicuspid aortic valve.

There is a low volume pulse and a coarse ejection systolic murmur radiating to the neck. There is usually an ejection click and its presence should make you suspect the diagnosis. Ejection murmurs radiating to the neck are common in children and usually innocent. The murmur of aortic stenosis tends to be harsher and there may be the accompanying early diastolic murmur of aortic incompetence.

Investigations

The heart is often normal on radiography. Post-stenotic dilatation of the aorta is variable and the heart muscle hypertrophies concentrically inwards so that the heart size on the chest radiograph often appears normal (*Fig.* 7.7).

The ECG is a relatively insensitive index of left ventricular hypertrophy in children but may show left ventricular hypertrophy. The echocardiogram may show concentric left ventricular thickening and restricted valve opening. The bicuspid nature of the valve may be identified.

It sometimes requires cardiac catheterization to determine the pressure gradient across the valve and hence the severity of the stenosis.

If this is greater than 50–70 mmHg aortic valvotomy should be performed. With lesser but significant degrees of aortic stenosis some restriction should be placed on the child's physical activities. We usually advise them to avoid competitive or demanding sports, e.g. jogging is all right but sprinting is not.

Subvalvular aortic stenosis

In addition to valvular aortic stenosis the narrowing may occur below the valve (subvalvular aortic stenosis). The subvalvular variety tends to be due to

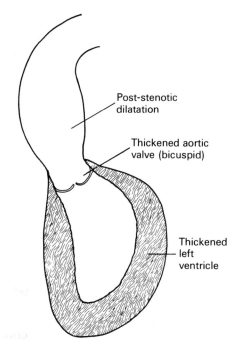

Post-stenotic dilatation

Thickened aortic valve (bicuspid)

Thickened left ventricle

Fig. 7.7.   Features of aortic stenosis.

inappropriately hypertrophied cardiac muscle which clamps down on itself during systole rather like a clenched fist. It is a variety of cardiomyopathy and when patients are symptomatic in childhood from this the outlook is poor. There is no ejection click and the aortic valve appears normal on the echocardiogram although it may close early. Occasionally subvalvular aortic stenosis is due to an intraventricular diaphragm.

Supravalvular aortic stenosis

Supravalvular aortic stenosis is rare There is usually narrowing of a relatively long portion of the aorta above the normal aortic valve. There is no ejection click and some cases run in families. Many cases are associated with infantile hypercalcaemia syndrome and there may be mental deficiency in this type. In all cases stenoses in the peripheral pulmonary arteries may also occur.

Aortic incompetence

This occasionally occurs in children either associated with aortic stenosis or on its own. Every effort is made to keep these children going to an age where they can have an adult size valve inserted. The majority, however, are asymptomatic and the heart can compensate for aortic incompetence for many years or even decades. In some cases of high ventricular septal defect the aortic valve leaflet may be able to prolapse downwards because of the lack of support. When the VSD is repaired the aortic reflux may be greatly improved.

Coarctation of the aorta

Clinical presentation

This is a fairly common form of congenital heart disease and like aortic stenosis may present early in life with heart failure or be picked up later on routine examination. The aorta is narrowed usually just distal to the left subclavian artery (*Fig*. 7.8) and hence the peripheral pulses in the upper and lower limbs are different in quality. The femoral pulses may be delayed and weak in comparison with the radials. In babies in heart failure where the femoral arteries cannot be felt coarctation of the aorta should be assumed to be present until proven otherwise.

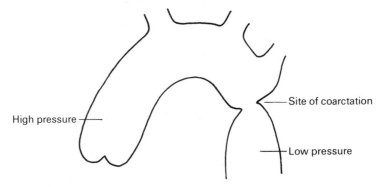

Fig. 7.8.   Coarctation of the aorta.

The more usual presentation is later in life when a murmur is heard on routine examination or the blood pressure in the upper limbs is found to be high and the femoral arteries are examined (often the presentation in young adults). The patients are usually symptom-free but death occurs, untreated, in the fourth decade largely from the consequences of high blood pressure. Collateral vessels carry blood from the pre-coarctation aorta to the post-coarctation aorta. Associated anomalies which occur are bicuspid aortic valve with variable degrees of stenosis, mitral incompetence and intracranial aneurysms in the circle of Willis. Even after correction of the coarctation surgically the risk of cerebral haemorrhage remains substantially higher than in the general population.

On examination the heart may be enlarged clinically and radiologically and the hum of blood flow through the large superficial collaterals may be heard especially at the back around the scapulae. These vessels may be palpable here. The femoral pulses are low volume and delayed or even absent. There is upper limb hypertension usually limited to the systolic and mean pressures with the diastolic more or less equal to that in the lower limb. An ejection systolic murmur may be heard especially radiating through to the back. Occasionally, an ejection click is heard and it can therefore be virtually impossible to tell clinically if there is associated aortic stenosis or not.

Chest radiograph

Classic appearances have been described on the chest radiograph. These are more apparent in the older child. Notching of the underside of the ribs occurs due to the large intercostal collaterals eroding the ribs. This is not usually seen before the age of 4 years. Two distinct bulges in the aorta may be seen each corresponding to the aorta pre- and post-coarctation. This is described as the '3' sign while with a barium swallow the exact opposite ('reverse 3 or E') sign may be seen in the oesophagus due to pressure on this structure from the aorta.

Surgery

In neonates not responding to anti-failure treatment the coarctation has to be resected. Apart from these cases there is some debate as to the timing of corrective surgery. Most would do this before school age but there has been a move recently to earlier correction about the age of 1 year. This is said to diminish the risk of developing sustained hypertension in later life which is about 50 per cent when the operation is performed pre-school. Some cases have recently been successfully treated by balloon dilatation but it remains to be seen how effective this is in the long term.

Preductal coarctation

A rare form of coarctation is when the narrowing occurs before the level of the ductus arteriosus. This is seen in neonates and is called preductal or infantile coarctation. Blood passes through the ductus to cause differential cyanosis of the lower limbs and there are usually other extensive cardiac abnormalities.

Left heart lesions

Other rare forms of acyanotic congenital heart disease affecting the left heart are mitral stenosis, mitral regurgitation, cor triatriatum (a diaphragm in the left atrium) and various anomalies of the aortic arch and great vessels such as aberrant subclavian arteries, aortic rings, etc.

Pulmonary stenosis

Clinical presentation

This is a relatively common form of congenital heart disease and may be valvular (the usual form) or infundibular where the stenosis is below the valve in the right ventricular outflow tract. Supravalvular pulmonary stenosis is very rare. Neonates may present with severe pulmonary stenosis and right heart failure and the differentiation from pulmonary atresia (unformed pulmonary valve) can be very difficult. More usually the abnormality is detected in the course of a routine medical examination. There is an ejection systolic murmur at the pulmonary area which radiates out clearly to the back. This finding of a well conducted murmur to the lung bases is a useful method of confirming that pulmonary stenosis is present. There is usually a thrill in the 2nd left intercostal space. There may be an ejection click with valvular stenosis although not with infundibular stenosis. The pulmonary second sound is widely split, may appear fixed, and the second component is soft. This splitting has been found to be in proportion to the degree of stenosis (*Fig.* 7.9). Thus, if at phonocardiography, the aortic and pulmonary components are 60 ms apart then the right ventricular pressure is 60 mmHg and so on for other values.

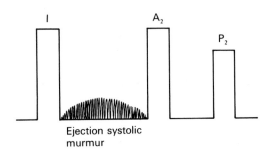

Fig. 7.9.   Heart sounds and murmur in pulmonary stenosis.

With significant valvular pulmonary stenosis the right ventricle and its outflow tract hypertrophy and so infundibular stenosis can be superimposed on valvular stenosis (*Fig.* 7.10).

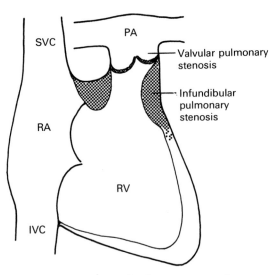

Fig. 7.10.   Types of pulmonary stenosis.

Investigations
The ECG may show right ventricular hypertrophy and right atrial hypertrophy.

The chest radiograph usually shows post-stenotic dilatation of the main pulmonary artery. The heart may sometimes be enlarged but usually the pulmonary vasculature is normal or diminished (a useful point in separating pulmonary stenosis from an ASD, both of which, as can be seen, are readily confused).

Echocardiography clearly distinguishes between the two and separates valvular from subvalvular stenosis.

As with aortic stenosis a gradient at cardiac catheterization of 50–70 mmHg at rest is required before performing pulmonary valvotomy or nowadays pulmonary valvuloplasty if the lesion is at the valve level.

With infundibular stenosis the right ventricular outflow tract needs to be reconstructed and the obstruction removed. This form of pulmonary stenosis is common with Fallot's tetralogy as will be discussed later.

Ebstein's anomaly
This constitutes about 1 per cent of congenital heart disease. The essential abnormality is that the tricuspid valve is seated lower than normal down in the right ventricle so that part of the ventricular muscle is, in fact, above the valve and incorporated in the right atrium (*Fig.* 7.11). The valve is abnormally formed and so also may be the remaining portion of the right ventricle to a variable extent. There is a whole spectrum of abnormalities but the crucial factor is just how much functioning right ventricle is present.

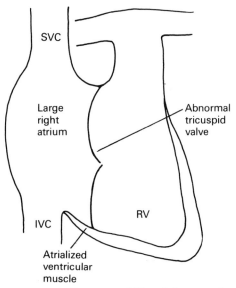

Fig. 7.11. Features of Ebstein's anomaly.

Right atrial pressure usually rises and there is also usually an ASD or patent foramen ovale so that blood goes from right to left at atrial level and the patients are variably cyanosed. The right atrium may become gigantic leading to further tricuspid incompetence from the already abnormal valve and to a greatly increased tendency for atrial arrhythmias.

Clinical presentation
The patients present with early right heart failure if the lesion is severe. Later in life they may just have reduced exercise tolerance and a tendency to supraventricular arrhythmia. There is often little to find on clinical examination although cyanosis and finger clubbing may be seen. Tricuspid incompetence may be apparent and there is sometimes a mid diastolic murmur over the lower end of the sternum.

Investigations
The chest radiograph shows an enlarged (sometimes aneurysmal) right atrium and where the right ventricle is not pumping much blood to the pulmonary vessels the lung fields may appear oligaemic. The echocardiogram confirms the altered anatomy.

Like ostium primum atrial septal defects, Ebstein's anomaly is one condition where the ECG is almost diagnostic. There are large P waves because of the right atrial enlargement and there is right bundle branch block because of the abnormal ventricle. A longish P-R interval may be seen as may paroxysmal atrial tachyarrhythmias.

At cardiac catheterization the diagnosis is confirmed by using a catheter with both pressure and electrical recording facilities. Atrial pressure is recorded while a ventricular ECG is being obtained from the same place representing the atrialization of the ventricle.

Treatment is largely symptomatic of the heart failure and arrhythmias.

Other rare right-sided lesions include pulmonary incompetence (much more common with pulmonary hypertension or after pulmonary valvotomy), tricuspid stenosis, tricuspid incompetence and double chambered (usually due to a diaphragm) right ventricle.

Cyanotic congenital heart disease

Tetralogy of Fallot (Fig. 7.12)
After the first year of life this is the commonest form of cyanotic congenital heart disease.

The tetralogy comprises pulmonary stenosis, ventricular septal defect, right ventricular hypertrophy and overriding of the aorta. Where there is an atrial septal defect in addition the combination is known as Fallot's pentalogy.

The severity of the condition varies largely depending on the degree of pulmonary stenosis. If this is marked then little blood will pass to the lungs but instead blood will shunt from right to left and pass out through the ventricular

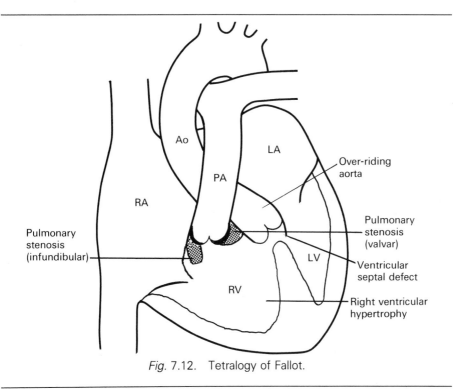

Fig. 7.12. Tetralogy of Fallot.

septal defect into the aorta. It is unusual for Fallot's tetralogy to be obvious at birth, usually taking some time to develop. The cyanosis tends to deepen as the child grows but may be intermittent only being apparent during cyanotic attacks or 'spells'. Infundibular as well as valvular pulmonary stenosis is often present and may become steadily worse.

Cyanotic spells

The cyanotic spells characteristic of this condition are thought to be due to spasm of the right ventricular outflow tract. Drugs, such as digoxin, which enhance myocardial contractility are to be avoided for this reason in patients with tetralogy of Fallot.

Cyanosis

Cyanosis is usually apparent with exertion or crying and either of these may be followed by a cyanotic spell. Cyanotic spells are emergencies and the child may lose consciousness and die. If such spells are occurring surgery is indicated even in otherwise pink children.

Squatting

Another characteristic feature of tetralogy of Fallot is squatting. The child squats frequently especially after exercise. This is thought to reduce blood flow to the legs and therefore to increase systemic resistance and decrease right to left shunting in the heart. They may also present with cerebral thrombosis or abscess.

On examination these patients are usually cyanosed. The heart is not usually much enlarged and there is the murmur of pulmonary stenosis. The ventricular septal defect contributes little to the murmurs because the pressures in the two ventricles are roughly equal except where the pulmonary stenosis is very mild (acyanotic tetralogy). A systolic thrill may be felt over the pulmonary area.

The chest radiograph is very helpful. The heart is classically 'boot shaped' with an upturned apex and relative absence of pulmonary arteries. The lung fields are usually oligaemic. The aortic arch is on the right side in 25–30 per cent and this may be the only abnormality detectable. The ECG reflects right ventricular hypertrophy. Echocardiography has been very useful and demonstrates the characteristic overriding of the aorta. Cardiac catheterization defines the anatomy for the surgeon and confirms the diagnosis.

Cyanotic spells have conventionally been treated with morphine. Beta-blocking drugs have been used more recently and these should be given prophylactically prior to surgery in those children having spells. Digoxin is to be avoided.

Surgery is initially palliative and takes the form of systemic artery to pulmonary artery shunting to allow the lung vessels to grow and to increase lung blood flow. Later on complete correction is indicated.

Other conditions causing cyanosis

Other rare forms of cyanotic congenital heart disease are pulmonary atresia with or without an associated ventricular septal defect, pulmonary stenosis with shunting at atrial level (right to left) and tricuspid atresia (severely malformed tricuspid valve). All of these have in common an inability of blood to pass to the lungs from the right ventricle and so cyanosis is early and marked in comparison with Fallot's tetralogy and the lung fields are oligaemic.

● Transposition of the great arteries

This is a very common form of neonatal congenital heart disease. Surgery for this lesion has improved dramatically in recent years and it is one of the growing points of paediatric cardiology. The positions of the two great arteries are reversed so that the aorta is now the anterior great vessel and connected to the right ventricle. Thus the systemic and pulmonary circulations are completely separate and unless some connection is established between them death willl ensue. Usually, of course, the ductus arteriosus fulfils this function initially and allows survival. Some mixing may occur through the foramen ovale and some infants have an associated ventricular septal defect.

Cyanosis is apparent within a few days of birth and this may come and go in intensity as the ductus opens and closes. If this is the suspected lesion the ductus can be kept patent with prostaglandins.

There is usually little to hear on examination although the second sound may be loud.

The ECG shows right ventricular enlargement.

The chest radiograph (in the classic case) shows a narrow pedicle due to the aorta and pulmonary artery being anteroposterior to one another. The heart resembles an egg on its side. Echocardiography is helpful and an intravenous injection of saline 'contrast echocardiography' will show the aorta filling before the pulmonary artery. On 2-D echocardiography there is a typical picture that establishes the diagnosis.

Cardiac catheterization is performed early and a hole is torn in the atrial septum by inflating a balloon full of contrast medium in the left atrium and then pulling it back to the right atrium. This is Rashkin's procedure (or atrial septostomy) and allows mixing of the two separate circulations.

Palliative shunts to the pulmonary artery or removal of the atrial septum can be performed later. Rastelli's, Mustard's and Senning's operations are all complex intra-atrial rearrangements to try and re-route blood to the appropriate vessel. More recently complete correction has been attempted. While this holds great promise for the future the surgical mortality is still very high.

When children have an associated ventricular septal defect (about 30 per cent) the presentation tends to be rather later, there is the murmur of a ventricular septal defect, and the heart is enlarged with failure. Atrial septostomy is still carried out and pulmonary artery banding performed if indicated. Later surgical correction is essentially similar to that performed in those infants without ventricular septal defects.

● Corrected transposition of the great arteries

Here there is unusual looping of the primitive heart tube of the embryo such that the end result is the right atrium connected to the left ventricle which itself is connected to the pulmonary artery. The left atrium connects to the right ventricle and then to the aorta. Thus the transposition has been 'corrected' but leaves the left ventricle pumping to the lungs and the right ventricle to the systemic circulation. The relationship of these vessels to each other is not, however, normal.

Not surprisingly such a scramble is associated with a very high incidence of other defects such as ventricular septal defects, pulmonary stenosis, 'mitral' incompetence and 'tricuspid' incompetence. The morphological right ventricle also finds it rather a struggle coping with the systemic load and arrhythmias are common.

● Persistent truncus arteriosus

This is a rare defect and several different types have been described. Basically the aorta and main pulmonary artery share a common 'truncal' valve and indeed these vessels may be the one structure. Cyanosis may be mild but heart failure is common. The pulses are often bounding and the lung fields plethoric; a clinical picture resembling a large ductus and indeed the murmur is also ejection systolic. The lesion carries a high risk both at surgery or if left untreated.

● Anomalous pulmonary venous drainage

In this defect blood returns from the lungs to the right atrium. It may be partial (usually the right upper pulmonary vein) or total and in some cases of total anomalous pulmonary venous drainage there is also obstruction to the return of blood to the right side so that pulmonary oedema develops. In total anomalous pulmonary venous drainage some connection is required between the right and left sides of the heart and usually this is via a patent foramen ovale.

The restricted forms present early in life with cyanosis and pulmonary congestion. The non-restricted forms present later with failure to thrive and cyanosis. In about half there are other cardiac abnormalities but in the isolated defect there are often no murmurs and the lesion and chest radiograph appearances can be almost indistinguishable from primary lung disease.

Cardiac catheterization may be needed to establish the diagnosis and to define the anatomy. Usually the pulmonary veins coalesce to form one large abnormal vessel which may join the right-sided circulation at a number of points either above or below the diaphragm. Fortunately at some point the vessel is closely related to the left atrium and the two can be connected surgically with ligation of the distal part.

There are many other complex forms of congenital heart disease such as anomalous coronary arteries, double outlet right ventricle, etc. A few general points are worth making.

Pulmonary artery banding

Where the lung fields are being flooded in large shunts pulmonary artery banding (creating an artificial pulmonary stenosis) often prevents heart failure and pulmonary hypertension.

Surgical shunts

Where pulmonary blood flow is poor this can be increased by systemic arterial to pulmonary artery shunting. This is necessary to get the pulmonary arteries to grow to allow for later correction. Examples of such shunts are Waterston (right pulmonary artery to ascending aorta); Blalock–Hanlon (removal of the atrial septum); Blalock–Taussig (right subclavian artery to right pulmonary artery); Potts (descending aorta to left pulmonary artery). Operative mortality under 6 months of age even for simple procedures is high, hence the need for palliation.

Hyperoxic test

The hyperoxic test is useful in deciding whether cyanosis is due to congenital heart disease or not. Breathing pure oxygen ought to raise the arterial P_{O_2} to at least 150 mmHg in non-cardiac hypoxia. This is a useful test especially in suspected anomalous pulmonary veins.

Prostaglandins and indomethacin

In cases with absent valves or no connection between the two circulations (pulmonary atresia; transposition of the great vessels) prostaglandin E_1 or E_2 will keep the ductus arteriosus open and buy time. In premature infants between the age of 28–40 weeks indomethacin either orally or intravenously may antagonize endogenous prostaglandins and cause a patent ductus to close.

Eisenmenger's syndrome

When patients with left to right shunts, e.g. VSD, ASD and patent ductus, develop pulmonary hypertension the shunt eventually reverses and becomes right to left. This is called Eisenmenger's syndrome and when this develops surgical intervention is no longer possible.

8

Coronary artery disease

One of the astonishing changes in medicine in this century is the extraordinary rise in the incidence of coronary artery disease. Although angina pectoris was described by Heberden in 1768 and well reported thereafter a considerable number of these cases were due to syphilis. It was not until 1912 that it was first reported that a patient could sustain and survive a myocardial infarction although it is now well known that John Hunter, who described his own angina and died from it while raging at his technician, had a myocardial infarction some 20 years before his death. The textbooks were reluctant to take up myocardial infarction as a definite diagnosis until the 1950s. Sir Thomas Lewis' textbook (1948) barely mentions the subject. It quickly became apparent, however, that myocardial infarction was reaching epidemic proportions. At present it is estimated that approximately 150 000 patients a year die from the disease in the United Kingdom and 500 000 in the USA. It was not until the 1960s that coronary care units were developed to cope with the major complication of a myocardial infarction, i.e. arrhythmias. In 1944 Paul Dudley White had written 'such arrhythmias (ventricular ectopics) are usually of relatively little importance'. When ECGs were continuously recorded in the 1950s during the first few hours of a myocardial infarction it was realized that ventricular ectopics may lead on to ventricular tachycardia and ventricular fibrillation. Now, almost every general hospital has a coronary care unit.

● **Aetiology of atheroma**

Atheroma (Gk = porridge) appears to be laid down in the coronary arteries as early as the late teens or early 20s with gradually increasing deposition occurring thereafter.

The cause of atheroma still remains a mystery and much attention has been focused on cholesterol which appears in quantity in the plaques along with platelets, fibrin and various white cells. A number of factors have been identified which may precipitate atheroma.

Major factors

1. *Age*
The incidence of ischaemic heart disease rises with age. The true incidence in the elderly is uncertain because the label 'ischaemic heart disease' may be applied without proper evidence. In coronary care units the numbers of patients admitted rises gradually up to the age of 70.

2. *Sex*
Under the age of 45 males are 10 times more likely to develop myocardial infarction than females. A striking increase in coronary artery disease occurs after the menopause in females. Whether oestrogens are responsible for this is unclear although it has been noted that premenopausal females have higher high density lipoprotein cholesterol and lower low density lipoprotein cholesterol. One very large study suggests that post-menopausal women taking oestrogens have half the risk of ischaemic heart disease events, fatal or non-fatal. Oestrogen in older men, e.g. stilboestrol for men with prostatic cancer, appears to increase the cardiovascular risk. It is not clear therefore why there is such a difference in the incidence of ischaemic heart disease between the sexes.

3. *Lipids*
During the Second World War the incidence of ischaemic heart disease fell in Scandinavia with its dietary deprivations compared with the United States. In the 1950s Ancel Keys published his study showing that the higher the average cholesterol in a particular country the higher the incidence of ischaemic heart disease. Japan had a very low incidence of heart disease with a low national average cholesterol while the reverse was true then for Finland. A subsequent study showed that Japanese people who had emigrated to the western United States rapidly increased their incidence of ischaemic heart disease suggesting diet as a factor. The Framingham study showed that in men aged 30–49 years there was a linear increase in mortality from ischaemic heart disease proportional to the serum cholesterol. In a major primary prevention trial in the USA, the Coronary Primary Prevention Trial, a 9 per cent reduction in cholesterol was associated with a 19 per cent reduction in fatal and non-fatal infarcts.

Cholesterol is fractionated into high density lipoproteins (HDL) and low density lipoproteins (LDL). High levels of HDL appear to be protective while high levels of LDL are closely related to high levels of ischaemic heart disease. It is important now to have these results and not just a total cholesterol. LDL is probably raised by saturated fatty acids in the diet (e.g. dairy products) while HDL can be raised by exercise and small amounts of alcohol (therefore run from pub to pub!). When fractionation is unavailable the level of total cholesterol is still helpful. A recent European consensus decided that we should aim to reach a level of 5.2 μmol/l in patients although accepted that this would mean almost 80 per cent of the population had high cholesterol. A figure of 6.5 μmol/l is accepted as the upper limit of normal and that all treatment should begin with diet. However, diet rarely drops the total cholesterol by more than about 10 per cent and drug treatment may be required particularly for levels above 7.5 μmol/l. The most useful group of drugs for treating hypercholesterolaemia at present are the HMG co-enzyme A reductase inhibitors, like simvastatin, which reduce the cholesterol by up to 30–50 per cent. Triglycerides are not as closely related to ischaemic heart disease as cholesterol but figures above 4–5 μmol/l need reducing by diet. Triglycerides rather than cholesterol are influenced by a recent meal so that a fasting blood lipid test is required, i.e. a blood test after 12–14 hours of a water-only diet.

4. *Smoking*
Smoking influences ischaemic heart disease by promoting atheroma. In general those who smoke 10 cigarettes per day double their risk of coronary heart disease, those who smoke 20 cigarettes per day treble their risk and those who smoke more than 20 cigarettes per day quadruple their risk. Filter cigarettes do not significantly alter the risk. Pipe and cigar smokers have only a slightly increased risk compared with non-smokers. Those who stop smoking undoubtedly decrease their coronary heart disease risk but even after 5 years it never quite equals those who do not smoke.

5. *Hypertension*
High blood pressure causes accelerated atheroma although the mechanism is unknown. Treatment of hypertension has reduced the incidence of stroke but not ischaemic heart disease. It has been suggested that this might be related to the treatment itself and possibly related to glucose intolerance induced by the drugs themselves. This remains to be proved.

Minor factors

1. *Exercise*
It is difficult, mainly due to methodological limitations, to prove that exercise prevents ischaemic heart disease. Indeed the cynic will state that jogging is positively dangerous with a significant mortality (road accidents, muggings, sudden cardiac death) and that the main feeling of wellbeing in sportsmen is merely the production of endorphins. Most physicians feel that exercise is of value and recommend that three times per week for a period of 20 minutes with enough exercise to make you breathless is helpful.

2. *Stress*
The difficulty with stress is that it is very difficult to measure its degree and the body's reaction to it. Plasma catecholamines rise with stress but other hormones

are involved. A sudden severe shock such as being in a car accident may be the last straw and result in a myocardial infarct. However, chronic stress is more difficult to assess. After periods of severe stress, e.g. divorce, death of a loved one or house moving, there is an increase in ischaemic heart disease episodes but precisely what part is played by stress is not known. Studies have suggested that the type 'A' personality, the hard driving, time-watching person is more likely to have coronary heart disease than the type 'B' personality who is easy going and less ambitious. While this may be true, there is not a great deal that can be done about one's personality.

3. *Obesity*
Despite the general public's idea that obesity is a great hazard, in fact, the patient has to be 20–30 per cent over his ideal body weight before an increased mortality can be registered.

3. *Alcohol*
Heavy alcohol consumption increases the incidence of ischaemic heart disease and hypertension. At one time it was reported that small amounts of alcohol were beneficial, possibly by raising the HDL cholesterol. Recent studies suggest this may not be true.

5. *Minerals*
Low copper levels, high zinc levels and soft water all may predispose, probably minimally, to ischaemic heart disease.

6. *Glucose intolerance*
Diabetics have a significant risk of ischaemic heart disease. About 2–6 per cent of the population have frank diabetes while another 20 per cent have impaired glucose tolerance. How significant this latter group is in terms of ischaemic heart disease is currently being investigated.

7. *Race*
A number of racial differences have been observed. The Japanese in Japan and the Black Africans in traditional surroundings have a very low incidence of ischaemic heart disease, while people of Asian origin tend to have a greater incidence of ischaemic heart disease compared with Caucasians and also to have larger myocardial infarctions.

● **Angina pectoris**
   Angina pectoris (angina = to strangle, pectoris = shoulder) describes symptoms related to a clinical situation. It therefore depends entirely on the patient's history. Angina pectoris is equated with the situation where retrosternal chest pain develops during exertion and goes away 2 or 3 minutes

after exercise ceases. It is worse in cold or windy weather or after meals and may develop during periods of emotion or excitement (e.g. an enthusiast watching an exciting sport). It does not develop *after* exercise, it does not last a long time after exercise except in exceptional circumstances and it is not accompanied necessarily by other symptoms, e.g. fatigue, dyspnoea or palpitations. These symptoms may occur in the patient but are not implicit in the term angina pectoris. The chest pain may radiate to the right arm or both arms, to the jaw and teeth, to the neck and occasionally to the back. In some instances, the chest pain may be absent and the patient may present with pain in the left arm only or even go to the dentist with toothache on exertion.

Angina is usually caused by a narrowing of the coronary arteries resulting in an imbalance of oxygen supply and demand but in a few cases spasm of the coronary arteries may occur. Angina can also be caused by aortic stenosis and rarely by hypertrophic cardiomyopathy. Occasionally, typical angina may occur without any demonstrable lesion of either the coronary arteries or the structure of the heart. This has been labelled 'syndrome X'.

Diagnosis

The diagnosis of angina pectoris is made primarily on the history. Attention must be paid to obtaining a precise account of the pain. Despite this there are a number of occasions when the history is of chest pain but a definite diagnosis cannot be made. In such a situation the following tests may be helpful.

1.   *Resting ECG*

Signs of ischaemia are:

a.   T wave changes (particularly inversion) over a number of leads are often diagnostic of ischaemia. T wave inversion in leads II, III, aVF = inferior ischaemia.

T wave inversion $V_2 - V_6$ = anterior ischaemia.

Note that T wave inversion in leads III, aVF and V_1 is common and does not necessarily imply ischaemia.

b.   Tall, pointed and symmetrical T waves may represent ischaemia.

c.   Inverted U waves (small waves following the T waves, best seen in $V_2 - V_4$) are suggestive of ischaemia.

d.   ST segment depression.

e.   T wave taller in V_1 than V_6.

2.   *Exercise ECG*

This is not an easy test to perform. It can either be achieved by the two-step test described by Masters or using a treadmill.

The Masters two-step test

The patient runs or walks up and down two fairly small steps (*Fig.* 8.1) until he is tired or develops symptoms. An ECG is taken before the test, may be monitored during the test and is taken in full after the test. Its drawback is that the amount of work done is not standardized and it is difficult to tell when the patient has done enough exercise.

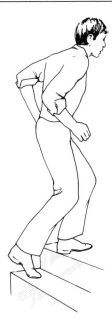

Fig. 8.1.   Two-step exercise test.

Treadmill (Fig. 8.2).

The treadmill test is a more reliable indicator of the amount of exercise a patient can perform. Every 3 minutes the speed and slope of the treadmill increase while the ECG is being monitored. Finally, the patient is walking at 5 m.p.h. up an 18° slope. A bicycle ergometer may be used instead.

Observations during an exercise test

Symptoms

If chest pain develops the patient should describe it and should be asked if it disappears when the exercise stops. Symptoms such as fatigue, dyspnoea or palpitations should be noted.

ECG

ST segment depression and ectopic beats and other ECG arrhythmias suggest coronary artery disease. The maximal heart rate is important. Unless activity is taken to a maximum the test may not be positive. A heart rate of 150+ should be achieved in most patients if possible. (A useful guide is 220 beats/min minus the subject's age.)

Blood pressure

A marked fall in blood pressure between the beginning and the end of the tests suggests significant coronary artery disease.

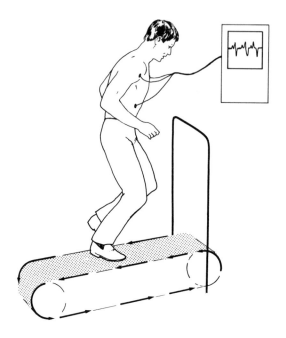

Fig. 8.2.   Treadmill exercise test.

3.   *Radioisotope studies*

Thallium-201 uptake during angina (or even at rest) is much reduced over the area of ischaemia giving a cold spot on the picture. This can be a useful test for angina but is expensive to set up and run. It is usually done during exercise to increase the sensitivity of the test.

4.   *Coronary angiography*

In cases where there is an absolute need for diagnosis of puzzling chest pain (e.g. airline pilots) coronary angiography can define areas of severe narrowing which are presumed to cause his angina.

Management

1.   *Mild angina*

a.   Explanation

It is very important for the patient to understand his angina and how to cope with it.

b.   Activities

The patient should avoid activities which bring on angina, e.g. rushing up stairs. He might be well advised to stroll to the railway or bus station rather than be late and have to rush.

c.   Stop smoking.

d.   Reduce emotional stress by tranquillizers if necessary.

e.   Weight reduction
Obesity increases the work load of the heart so that increased exercise tolerance will occur if weight loss is achieved.

f.   Glyceryl trinitrate (GTN)
This is useful for relieving anginal pain if taken correctly. GTN lasts about 30 minutes and may take up to 2–3 minutes for its action to start. There is less point, therefore, in taking it after the pain has developed because when you stop to suck the tablet the pain will start to disappear in 2–3 minutes anyway. It is ideally taken before exercise so as to increase the amount of work that can be done before pain starts. GTN is dissolved under the tongue and is colloquially known as TNT, particularly as its main side effect is a pounding headache. Patients should be told to swallow the tablet (rendering it inactive) at a time before it causes the headache (e.g. 90 s). It can also be given by sublingual spray.

g.   Treat congestive cardiac failure if present.

h.   Treat hypertension and arrhythmias if present.

2.   *Moderate angina*

Management of moderate angina includes the points mentioned above in mild angina but in addition:

Beta-blockers

Beta-blockers are drugs which are both negatively chronotropic as well as negatively inotropic. On both counts there is a reduction in O_2 consumption and thus a relief of angina. The patient's heart rate will usually drop to around 60 but the important test is the rise in heart rate on exercise. Only if the heart rate barely alters is the patient fully beta-blocked and therefore deriving maximum benefit. A short walk when the patient visits the outpatient department is sufficient to demonstrate this fact. Any beta-blocker will have this effect but the 'cardioselective' agents (e.g. atenolol, metoprolol) may have fewer side effects.

Calcium antagonists

These drugs which prevent the normal movement of calcium in the myocardium 'uncouple' electrical and mechanical contraction and so reduce oxygen consumption. Nifedipine, diltiazem and verapamil can be used, very often successfully, either alone or in combination with other anti-anginal agents. Beta-blockers and verapamil together are best avoided. Nifedipine may have the added advantage of preventing coronary artery spasm. There are newer calcium antagonists becoming available which may confer additional advantages.

Long-acting nitrates

Because GTN only lasts about 30 minutes a long-acting nitrate would be very advantageous to the patient. The dinitrates are metabolized rapidly by the liver, the 'first pass' effect, and are poorly absorbed. Nonetheless, they are at least partly effective. The mononitrates do not suffer from the 'first pass' effect and do appear to be helpful. It is important however to allow a nitrate-free period every 24 hours, to allow the drug to be most effective. GTN is destroyed by the liver and therefore is unsuitable for oral use but it can be absorbed through the skin. There are proprietary GTN patches which can be used, therefore, to get a steady blood level over prolonged periods.

3.   *Severe angina*

When the patient is on triple therapy (beta-blockers, calcium antagonists and nitrates) angiography should be considered if the following conditions apply.

a.   Failed medical therapy

   (i)   The angina is still very limiting despite triple therapy.

  (ii)   The angina is controlled but only at the expense of unacceptable side effects of the medication, e.g. the 'weariness and dreariness' of beta-blockers.

b.   Young patients (< 45 years).

If angiography demonstrates significant narrowing, intervention must be considered.

a.   Angioplasty

A balloon is introduced into the coronary artery across the narrowing and inflated. This procedure is repeated as often as is necessary. The narrowing is reduced by squeezing fluid out of the atheroma or by forcing the atheroma along the media of the coronary artery rather like toothpaste. Its proper name is percutaneous transluminal coronary angioplasty (PTCA).

The balloon is introduced into the artery using X-ray control. At the time of angioplasty 2–4 per cent of patients will urgently require coronary artery bypass grafting because of damage to the artery.

While this procedure is not perfect and is limited to reasonably accessible lesions of the arteries it is usually performed in preference to coronary artery bypass grafting (CABG) if possible. It is much less traumatic and will only involve the patient in a 3-day inpatient stay.

b.   Coronary artery bypass grafting (*Fig.* 8.3)

If angioplasty is not possible, the narrowings of the artery are bypassed using saphenous vein sutured to the base of the aorta and to the coronary

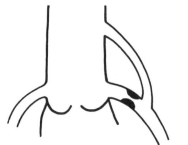

Fig. 8.3.   Coronary artery bypass graft.

artery distal to the lesion. The internal mammary arteries can also be used to provide up to two grafts.

There are three factors which might be influenced by this procedure.

a. Chest pain, i.e. angina. The operation is highly successful for chest pain, relieving it completely in 60–70 per cent of cases and making an improvement in a further 25 per cent or so. Up to 95 per cent of patients thus derive benefit. There is, however, a recurrence rate of 50 per cent in about 10 years, albeit not necessarily severe.

b. Life span. So far, life span has only been shown to be clearly improved in two situations – left main stem disease (*Fig.* 8.4a) and triple vessel disease (*Fig.* 8.4b). Left main stem disease is known as 'the widow maker' and

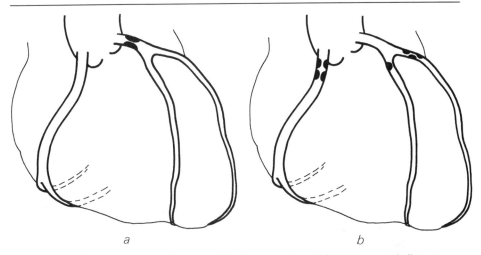

Fig. 8.4. Coronary artery disease. (a) Left main stem. (b) Triple vessel disease.

surgery improves life expectancy at 5 years by 30 per cent (*Fig.* 8.5). Surgery improves triple vessel disease at 5 years by 10–15 per cent (*Fig.* 8.6). No clear difference in survival has so far appeared in single or double vessel disease.

c. Left ventricular function. No study has shown any consistent improvement in left ventricular function, although this undoubtedly occurs in some individual cases.

Coronary artery bypass grafting remains an operation for relief of chest pain in the majority of cases. Younger patients may deserve earlier consideration for coronary angiography in case they have left main stem disease. This syndrome may be suspected during a treadmill exercise test by:

a. ST depression of 4 mm appearing rapidly.

b. Large drop in blood pressure during exercise.

c. Onset of arrhythmias after minimal exertion.

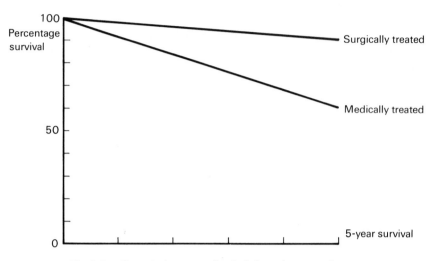

Fig. 8.5.   Cumulative mortality in left main stem disease.

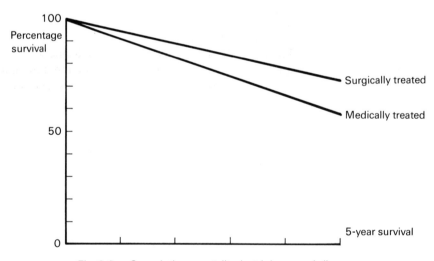

Fig. 8.6.   Cumulative mortality in triple vessel disease.

Prognosis of angina pectoris

The overall mortality of the group is about 4 per cent per year. Factors which adversely affect the prognosis are:

a.   Uncontrolled hypertension (>150/90).

b.   Congestive cardiac failure.

c.   Previous myocardial infarction.
d.   Number of coronary arteries affected.
According to the Framingham study, one-quarter of male patients with angina will have an infarct within 5 years (one-eighth in women) and one-third will die in 8 years.

● **Unstable angina**
'Unstable', 'crescendo' or 'preinfarction' angina are synonymous names which describe a variety of syndromes in which chest pain occurs at rest without evidence of infarction but which may be followed immediately or after further bouts of pain by a full myocardial infarction. Many of the patients will have known angina of effort and the sudden change must be taken seriously. Myocardial infarction does not always follow, but it may do so and efforts to reduce the risk of infarction must be taken immediately.

1.   *Medical*
A reduction in myocardial oxygen demand is essential and can be achieved by:
a.   A beta-blocker (e.g. atenolol)
b.   A calcium antagonist (e.g. nifedipine)
c.   A nitrate (e.g. isosorbide mononitrate).
Either all three drugs can be used or any number in combination. In addition aspirin is used as an anticoagulant and has proved to be very beneficial. Using this regimen around 85 per cent of patients with this syndrome will settle and can be discharged from hospital on suitable therapy. In the remaining patients the chest pain does not settle and further measures should be considered.

2.   *Surgical*
If medical therapy fails, coronary angiography followed by coronary artery bypass grafting or angioplasty may be life saving.
Whatever the therapy, ultimately between 15–30 per cent of all patients will develop a myocardial infarction.

● **Myocardial infarction**
Myocardial infarction is now the commonest mode of death in western countries. The precise mechanism by which the blockage of a coronary artery occurs is not known. Several theories have been suggested (*Fig.* 8.7):
1.   Thrombosis occurs in an already atheromatous vessel.
2.   Bleeding occurs into an atheromatous plaque which has ruptured as a result of pressure.
3.   Spasm of the coronary artery obliterates the lumen.

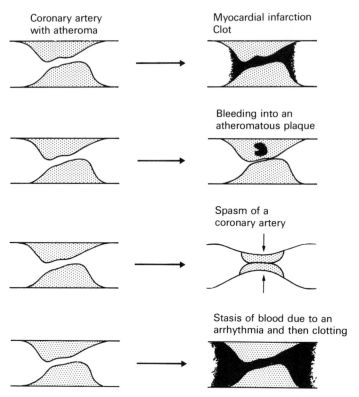

Coronary artery with atheroma

Myocardial infarction Clot

Bleeding into an atheromatous plaque

Spasm of a coronary artery

Stasis of blood due to an arrhythmia and then clotting

Fig. 8.7.   Possible pathological sequelae of coronary artery atheroma.

4.   Onset of a tachyarrhythmia may make the heart ischaemic when the vessels are already atheromatous and stasis of blood in the lumen may lead to thrombosis.

Symptoms
Prodromal symptoms of a myocardial infarction are not common but in retrospect many patients complain of tiredness for weeks or months beforehand. A relatively small proportion have angina pectoris and then develop a myocardial infarction.

The predominant symptom of a myocardial infarction is chest pain (*Fig.* 8.8). The chest pain is typically retrosternal, very severe, crushing in nature and radiating to the left arm and neck. The patient often feels a sense of suffocation and impending death. With the pain comes nausea, sweating and a feeling of cold. Occasionally dizziness and collapse occur, particularly if the pain causes a vasovagal response. If the infarct is large, left ventricular failure may develop with dyspnoea and occasionally pink frothy sputum (pulmonary oedema).

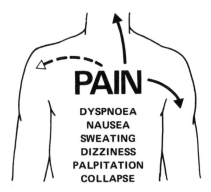

Fig. 8.8.   The symptoms of myocardial infarction.

Signs

The signs of a myocardial infarction are disappointingly few. Unless a complication (e.g. left ventricular failure) has developed the heart will probably be normal to examination. The complications which may develop and produce physical signs soon after the infarction begins to evolve are as follows.

1.   *Left ventricular failure*

Crepitations at the lung bases. Gallop rhythm (third or fourth heart sound). Pulsus alterans (very rare indeed).

2.   *Cardiogenic shock (extreme left ventricular failure)*

Hypotension (systolic 80 mmHg or less). Patient looks grey, cold and sweaty. Urine output ceases.

3.   *Rupture of*

a.   Free wall of left ventricle – signs of cardiac tamponade.

b.   Mitral cusp – loud pansystolic murmur over mitral area radiating to axilla with signs of left ventricular failure.

c.   Ventricular septum – harsh pansystolic murmur over left sternal edge with signs of left ventricular failure.

4.   *Pericarditis*

Pericardial friction rub. Raised ST segments on ECG.

5.   *Systemic emboli*

Signs of ischaemia in limbs with severe pain. Signs of a stroke.

6.   *Pulmonary emboli*

Pleuritic chest pain. Pleural rub. If large, cyanosis and collapse.

Diagnosis

A strong suspicion of the diagnosis is obvious from the history but 3 per cent of normal patients and up to 20 per cent of diabetic patients may have no chest pain. Even short episodes of chest pain must not be dismissed.

As soon as any suspicion of a myocardial infarction is aroused an ECG must be performed.

1.   *The ECG*

A wide variety of changes in the ECG may suggest myocardial infarction but there is a classic pattern of a full infarct which evolves. In the first few hours after an infarction the ECG may be normal, then the ST segment rises (*Fig*. 8.9):

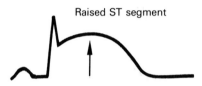

Raised ST segment

Fig. 8.9.   The ECG of acute stage of a myocardial infarction (first few hours).

Then develops the 'full blown' pattern of myocardial infarction (*Fig*. 8.10). After a few more hours (up to 24 hours) the ST segment reverts to normal leaving a Q wave and inverted T wave. Because tissue death is a permanent change Q waves will usually be found long term in the patient's ECG but the T wave will often become upright post-infarction.

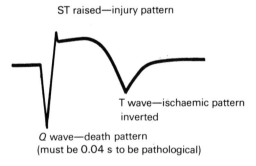

ST raised—injury pattern

T wave—ischaemic pattern
inverted

Q wave—death pattern
(must be 0.04 s to be pathological)

Fig. 8.10.   The ECG in the later stages of myocardial infarction.

It is unwise to expect those changes in every patient and the appearances in some patients may only be T wave inversion or peaking of the T waves (subendocardial infarction) (*Fig*. 8.11) or nothing at all when the diagnosis must be made by other means.

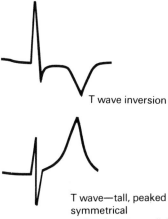

T wave inversion

T wave—tall, peaked
symmetrical

Fig. 8.11.   ECG patterns of subendocardial infarction.

Site of infarction
It is useful to locate the site of a myocardial infarction because the pattern of the illness is slightly different.

Anterior: Large muscle loss – therefore most likely to develop left ventricular failure.

Tachycardia (large muscle loss).

Inferior: Bradycardia common (? vagal response).

Heart block more likely – the AV node is supplied in 90 per cent (approx.) by the right coronary artery.

Ruptured mitral valve cusp more common.

The site of the myocardial infarction is made by observing the leads in which the changes have occurred (*Figs.* 8.12 and 8.13).

Leads I and aVL observe the anterolateral aspect of the heart and may show changes in an anterior myocardial infarction.Leads II, III, and AV$_F$ observe the inferior surface.

2.   *Enzymes*
The sudden death of tissue releases enzymes from the cells. In myocardial infarction, creatinine phosphokinase (CPK), alanine serum transaminase (AST – formerly known as serum glutamic oxalotransaminase – SGOT) and lactic dehydrogenase (LDH) are released in abundance and their rise and subsequent fall is used to diagnose an infarction (*Fig.* 8.14).

These enzymes are not unique to cardiac muscle and therefore an event (the chest pain) followed by a rise and fall of enzyme is required for complete diagnosis. CPK can be released from skeletal muscle damage, LDH rises after a pulmonary embolus and AST in liver disease. Care must, therefore, be taken to interpret the results correctly and a single enzyme result may be valueless.

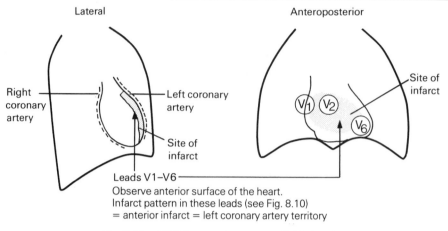

Observe anterior surface of the heart.
Infarct pattern in these leads (see Fig. 8.10)
= anterior infarct = left coronary artery territory

Fig. 8.12   ECG in anterior myocardial infarction.

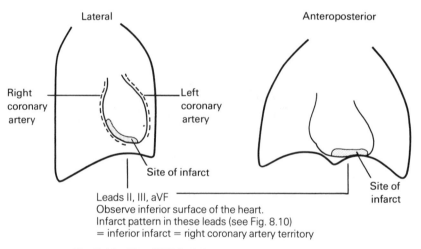

Observe inferior surface of the heart.
Infarct pattern in these leads (see Fig. 8.10)
= inferior infarct = right coronary artery territory

Fig. 8.13   The ECG in inferior myocardial infarction.

Ideally the MB-CPK enzyme (myocardial fraction) should be estimated because this is always almost exclusively cardiac in origin. Serum enzymes are usually taken for 3 successive days after a suspected myocardial infarction.

3.   *Temperature, white cell count and erythrocyte sedimentation rate (ESR)*
a.   Temperature. The typical pyrexia of an infarction is shown in *Fig.* 8.15.

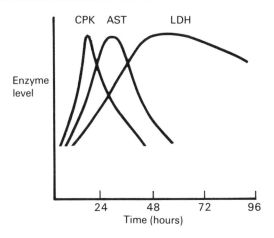

Fig. 8.14.   Patterns of enzyme rise and fall after myocardial infarction.

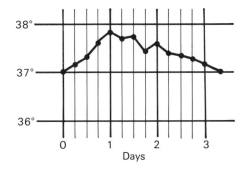

Fig. 8.15.   Pyrexia of myocardial infarction.

b.   A raised white cell count occurs after a myocardial infarction (above 11 500) and values above 20 000 indicate a poor prognosis.

c.   The ESR is often as high as 60–70.

4.   *Other tests*

Various radioisotopic studies have been performed, e.g. technetium-99m pyrophosphate is taken up by acutely necrosed myocardial tissue, but the apparatus is extremely expensive and the value of the tests in terms of an earlier diagnosis or measuring the size of the infarct have yet to be established (see chapter 4).

Management

One of the most significant advances to have been made in recent years is the understanding that thrombosis is the immediate cause of occlusion (and therefore of myocardial infarction) in atheromatous coronary vessels. More than 90 per cent of people dying from their infarct are found to have a thrombus at the site of vessel occlusion. This has led to the development of thrombolytic therapy which can re-open these thrombosed vessels and hence both prevent myocardial infarcts or limit their size. Streptokinase, anistreplase and tissue plasminogen activator (tPA) are the three thrombolytic agents in use. They each have advantages and disadvantages but streptokinase is by far the cheapest and is therefore the most widely used.

Thrombolytic agents have been shown to reduce the very early mortality by up to 50 per cent. They may still have advantages to confer if given up to 24 hours after an infarct but in general the sooner these drugs are administered then the greater the benefit. The use of early aspirin also seems to reduce mortality in its own right and adds to the benefits of streptokinase. It remains to be seen if aspirin is beneficial when used with the other agents or whether in the long term important differences emerge between thrombolytic agents.

One major complication of a myocardial infarction is an arrhythmia and this is the reason coronary care units (CCU) were established. The incidence of serious arrhythmias and sudden death is highest in the few hours immediately after a myocardial infarction. By 4 hours 60 per cent of the deaths following myocardial infarction have occurred. This means that the sooner the patient can reach hospital and the sooner the patient reaches the CCU the greater his chances of survival. This is especially true with the arrival of effective thrombolysis (*Fig.* 8.16).

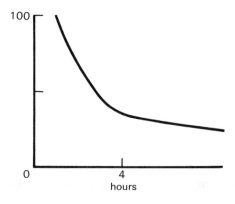

Fig. 8.16.   Percentage of deaths occurring post-infarction.

1.   *General management*
        Pain
Diamorphine i.v. or i.m. or both. Morphine causes venous pooling, a decrease in left ventricular filling pressure and decreased cardiac output. This may prevent impending left ventricular failure. Pethidine is a reasonable alternative but pentazocine is not recommended because it increases the left ventricular filling pressure and cardiac work.
        Sedation
Diazepam or equivalent is necessary for the very anxious patient but this will not usually be required. Sedation may also be needed for sleep particularly if the CCU is busy and there is a lot of noise at night.
        Nausea and vomiting
Fear and pain may produce vomiting as may diamorphine. Prochlorperazine or metoclopramide are used and cause no myocardial problems.
        Reassurance
It is better to inform a patient (except under special circumstances) as soon as you suspect an infarction rather than keeping him guessing.
        Anticoagulation
Although the subject of some debate, 5000 IU heparin three times daily appears to prevent the majority of both systemic and pulmonary emboli. This may be given subcutaneously. Its place following or with thrombolysis has yet to be fully evaluated.
        ECG monitor
An important aspect of the CCU is to deal with arrhythmias (see later).
        IV line
Direct access to a vein is of considerable importance. This can either be an indwelling needle flushed regularly with a small dose of heparin or a slowly running dextrose drip. Saline must be avoided as it may precipitate cardiac failure.
        Beta-blockade
Intravenous beta-blockade may be used – generally atenolol or metoprolol. In the absence of heart failure, heart block, etc. a bolus should be given as soon as possible. It reduces mortality possibly by limiting infarct size.

2.   *Treatment of complications*
        Arrhythmias
The diagnosis and management of arrhythmias are dealt with in chapter 9.
        Left ventricular failure (mild)
Diuretics as appropriate.
        Left ventricular failure (severe) – cardiogenic shock
When the systolic blood pressure falls below 100 mmHg and left ventricular failure begins to supervene the outlook becomes poor. The following actions may help:
    i. Infusion of inotropic agent, dopamine or dobutamine.
    ii. Diuretics.

   iii. Diamorphine to prevent agitation and distress.

   iv. Oxygen.

   v. Left atrial line. A balloon catheter floated into the pulmonary artery can be used to measure left atrial pressure. Occasionally the patient may have a low left ventricular filling pressure and can then be given dextrose to good effect.

   vi. Infusion of nitroprusside. Vasodilatation may offload the left ventricle and although may initially cause a small drop in pressure the cardiac output may rise and help the failure.

     This drug should only be used with careful monitoring of the arterial pressure.

   vii. Intra-aortic balloon pump (for details see chapter 5). Although patients may do well initially many die when the pump is switched off.

Systemic or pulmonary emboli

Full anticoagulation.

Pericarditis

Suggests a transmural infarction. No immediate treatment is necessary unless there is pain.

Sudden onset of pansystolic murmur

   i. Mitral incompetence (ruptured cusp). Heart failure will develop rapidly and must be treated. Valve replacement is ideally performed several weeks post-infarction and even then carries a high mortality but an intra-aortic balloon pump may 'buy' time very successfully.

   ii. Ventricular septal defect. Heart failure rapidly develops and the outlook is poor. Repair is possible ideally at about 6 weeks post-infarction but surgical mortality is high. Again, an intra-aortic balloon pump may 'buy' time.

     In both these cases timing of surgery is still controversial but seems to be moving towards earlier rather than later intervention.

Ventricular rupture

Death may occur instantaneously but occasionally a slow leak into the pericardium develops. This will present with pain and collapse. Echocardiography can diagnose this and pericardial aspiration may help but surgical repair may be necessary.

Post-myocardial infarction syndrome (Dressler's syndrome)

Chest pain associated with a pericardial friction rub developing weeks or months after a myocardial infarction is known as Dressler's syndrome. It is probably due to an autoimmune response against dead myocardial tissue and rapidly improves with steroids. If mild, indomethacin will suffice. There is a leucocytosis and often a fever.

     Most patients with a myocardial infarction will stay in the coronary care unit 2–3 days and in hospital a further 4–5 days. Complications will keep a patient in hospital longer but no specific benefit appears to be gained by keeping the patient in hospital for longer periods as used to be the case. When the patient goes home he must understand quite clearly what he can and cannot do. Here is a suggested regimen:

Week 1.   Pottering around the house only.
Week 2.   Pottering around the house and garden.
Week 3.   Pottering around house and garden and walking up to half a mile per day.
Week 4.   As in week 3 but walking 1 mile per day.
Weeks 5–8. Back to work part time then full time.

Prognosis

A figure of 15–18 per cent mortality in the first year and 7–9 per cent mortality thereafter is usually quoted but this appears to be falling, possibly to around 3–4 per cent per year, and presumably due to secondary prevention, and now to thrombolysis.

Factors suggesting a poor prognosis are:
1.   Large size of infarction.
2.   Previous infarction.
3.   Persistent angina, particularly if associated with ECG changes.
4.   Persistent arrhythmias.
5.   Cardiac arrest.
6.   Large heart on chest radiography (CTR > 50 per cent).
7.   Signs of left ventricular aneurysm.
8.   Persistent tachycardia.
9.   Left ventricular failure.

Secondary prevention (prevention of a further myocardial infarction)

This very important but somewhat neglected aspect of cardiology seems to be having a very positive effect upon prognosis after a myocardial infarction. There are two aspects:

Aspirin

Numerous secondary preventive trials, including those on transient ischaemic attacks, cerebrovascular accidents and intermittent claudication as well as myocardial infarction, have shown a reduction in mortality of 25 per cent using aspirin. All post-infarction patients, unless they have an active peptic ulcer, should take an aspirin a day. Any dose between 75 mg and 600 mg is acceptable.

Beta-blocker

Meta-analysis of all the beta-blocker trials shows a reduction at 1 year of 26 per cent in mortality (10.2 per cent *vs* 7.5 per cent). This benefit must be weighed against side effects, e.g. weariness and fatigue, impotence and left ventricular failure and therefore is usually introduced on an individual patient basis.

Other aspects of myocardial infarction

1. *Coronary care ambulance*

The high incidence of lethal arrhythmias in the first few hours following a myocardial infarction led to the introduction of coronary care ambulances. When a call is received by the ambulance centre that a patient has chest pain an ambulance equipped with cardiac monitoring and resuscitation equipment is rapidly directed to the scene. The ambulancemen are trained to deal with myocardial infarction and transfer the patient as quickly as possible to the coronary care unit. Results from the United States and Great Britain suggest that about 5 per cent of those patients collected by ambulance have lethal arrhythmias which they would not otherwise have survived. In future, thrombolytic agents may well be given by trained ambulance crews.

2. *Post CCU monitoring*

Suggestions that patients should be closely monitored in the days after their stay in the coronary care unit do not seem to be borne out in fact. No appreciable drop in mortality occurs because in the week following the stay in the CCU patients die predominantly from heart failure and not arrhythmias.

3. *Home or hospital care of the coronary patient*

Critics of CCUs suggest that the fear of being admitted to hospital increases the catecholamines to such an extent that the good a CCU achieves is offset by artificially induced arrhythmias. Three English studies (Newcastle, Bristol and Nottingham) have shown no difference in mortality between patients treated at home or in hospital. However, the studies have received much criticism because of their small numbers, large number of excluded patients and the 'drop-out' rate of patients from the study who developed complications at home and were thus admitted to hospital.

4. *Rehabilitation*

Most hospitals now run rehabilitation courses for post-infarct patients. They take the form of exercise programmes, psychological counselling or both. These courses are effective at reducing morbidity. A greater proportion of people counselled return to normal lives when compared with those discharged from care with no further counselling. There is recent evidence suggesting that rehabilitation may improve prognosis.

9

Arrhythmias

Arrhythmias are common problems. They may occur in people with entirely normal hearts or they may represent the clinical manifestation of serious cardiac disease. Being mainly intermittent they can present a formidable diagnostic challenge. Recent years have seen rapid therapeutic advances in the treatment of arrhythmias both fast and slow, so that great clinical satisfaction can be obtained from their treatment. Equally they may be refractory to practically every drug or manoeuvre and prove to be most frustratingly resistant to treatment.

There are two broad group of arrhythmias – fast and slow. Things are never that simple, of course, and there is a third group where both fast and slow arrhythmias may alternate (*Table* 9.1).

● Tachyarrhythmias

These are arrhythmias that are associated with a fast heart rate. For convenience isolated supraventricular and ventricular ectopic beats are usually included in this group. The patients often experience rapid palpitations, i.e. an awareness of the heart beating rapidly although many instances have been recorded on 24-hour ECGs where the patient has been completely oblivious to the fact and felt well. If the arrhythmia lasts for any length of time the patient usually becomes aware of something unusual occurring in the end. Fatigue is a common symptom as is dyspnoea and light-headedness, but actual loss of consciousness or syncope occurs less often. A good way to get an idea of what the arrhythmia is like is to get the patient to tap out on the desk with one finger his impression of the heart's rhythm. If the arrhythmia starts suddenly (switches on, is absent one second and present the next) a true arrhythmia is likely to be present and a sinus tachycardia is most unlikely. This is a most helpful symptom and should always be asked about. Myocardial excitants such as the caffeine in tea or coffee, alcohol or cigarette smoke tend to precipitate supraventricular

Table 9.1. Common arrhythmias

Tachyarrhythmias
  Sinus tachycardia
  Supraventricular ectopic beats
  Paroxysmal supraventricular tachycardia (SVT)
  Paroxysmal supraventricular tachycardia with block
  Atrial flutter
  Atrial fibrillation (AF)
  Pre-excitation syndromes (WPW)
  Ventricular ectopic beats
  Parasystole
  Ventricular tachycardia (VT)
  Ventricular fibrillation (VF)

Tachycardia-bradycardia syndrome (*sick sinus syndrome*)

Bradyarrhythmias
  Sinus bradycardia
  Sinus arrest
  Sino-atrial block
  First-degree heart block
  Second-degree heart block
    Mobitz Type I or Wenckebach
    Mobitz Type II
  Third-degree heart block (complete heart block)

arrhythmias. Often there is no recognizable precipitating factor. If the patient passes urine after an episode of palpitations then it is likely that he has had an arrhythmia. This is called urina spastica and is thought to be mediated via atrial receptors.

Patients often find manoeuvres that help to terminate attacks especially of supraventricular arrhythmias. Typically they lie down (thereby reducing sympathetic tone) and they may take a drink of cold water or hold their breath in a self-learnt Valsalva manoeuvre (both of which increase vagal tone). These points in the history are further evidence in favour of a cardiac arrhythmia as is the knowledge that exercise or exertion may precipitate an attack.

Physical examination should be carried out looking for a possible aetiology of the tachyarrhythmia. Thyrotoxicosis or mitral stenosis may be present, both of which typically lead to disturbances in cardiac rhythm.

Sinus tachycardia
The normal range of heart rate is 50–100 beats/min. Above this rate sinus tachycardia is present such as is seen with exercise or excitement. It may occur in heart failure or other conditions where there is increased sympathetic tone as a normal physiological response.

Sinus arrhythmia is a variant of sinus rhythm. The heart rate varies with respiration, increasing with inspiration (*Fig.* 9.1) and decreasing with expiration. It is seen in young people and tends to disappear with increasing age. The pulse irregularity may be quite marked.

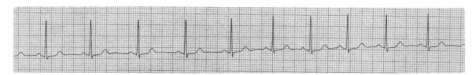

Fig. 9.1.   Sinus arrhythmia.

Supraventricular ectopic beats
Isolated beats arising from the atria but outside the sino-atrial node are common (*Fig.* 9.2). They are probably due to an ectopic excitable focus and are generally benign and do not need to be treated. Typically the P wave is abnormal although the PR interval is not. If very frequent the pulse may be quite irregular in which case the rhythm often goes on to one of the more established supraventricular arrhythmias.

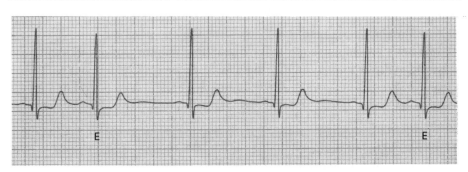

Fig. 9.2.   Atrial ectopic beats (E).

Paroxysmal supraventricular tachycardia
Bursts of regular atrial activity occur usually at a rate of about 140–180 beats/min. It may be faster, of course, and rates of up to 300/min are seen in young children and neonates without much apparent discomfort. In an adult, of course, such a rapid rate would cause acute distress. This arrhythmia is usually benign and the heart is basically healthy. It may be due to an ectopic focus in the atria but more often is due to a re-entry phenomenon. This simply means that the abnormal electrical impulse travels around the atria and by the time it returns to the point from which it started, the atrial muscle at this site is no

longer refractory and the abnormal wave can set off once more passing around the atrial muscle. It seems many of these 're-entry' tachycardias (and they can be seen in the ventricle too) are originating in or near the atrioventricular (AV) node itself (*Fig.* 9.3).

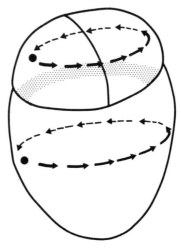

Fig. 9.3.   Mechanism of re-entry tachyarrhythmias.

The attacks are often self-limiting although they can go on for days. The patient has to decide whether prophylactic drug therapy is more of a nuisance than the arrhythmia itself. If the circulation is compromised in any way, e.g. hypotension, syncope, angina, etc., then treatment is indicated on safety grounds for what is basically otherwise a benign condition. Usually there is one P wave for every QRS complex but the P waves are somewhat abnormal and may be inverted in leads where usually they would be upright (e.g. lead I) (*Fig.* 9.4).

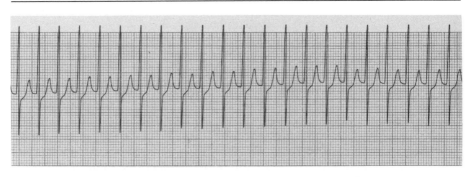

Fig. 9.4.   Paroxysmal supraventricular tachycardia.

The attack can often be terminated by a Valsalva manoeuvre, carotid sinus massage or a cold drink. These can be done at home either by the patient or his general practitioner. In hospital facial immersion in cool water is sometimes used. This evokes a vestigial diving response and induces marked vagal tone which may terminate the attack. Small amounts of a pressor agent such as phenylephrine may raise the blood pressure and cause a baroreflex-mediated vagal discharge. However, most physicians, if the non-invasive techniques do not work, inject one of the specific anti-arrhythmic agents. Verapamil slowly intravenously in a dose of up to 20 mg is usually effective. Seldom does one need a dose as large as this especially if carotid sinus massage is used at the same time. Other drugs include disopyramide, beta-blocking agents and the neglected but often successful procainamide. It should be noted that asystole may be caused by the concurrent intravenous use of verapamil and a beta-blocker. This combination should be avoided.

Electrical cardioversion may rarely be needed. When back in sinus rhythm control may be obtained with any of the drugs above or even with digoxin.

Paroxysmal atrial tachycardia with block

This is essentially an extension of paroxysmal supraventricular tachycardia without block. It is mentioned separately here because the majority are due to digoxin toxicity. When this arrhythmia is seen on the electrocardiogram it should be assumed to be due to digoxin until proved otherwise (*Fig.* 9.5).

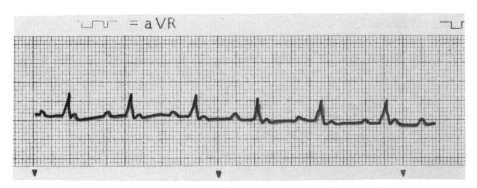

Fig. 9.5. Paroxysmal atrial techycardia with block.

Obviously this can be mistaken for 2:1 heart block but both the atrial and ventricular rates should be noted to be fast. Digoxin should be withdrawn and if the rhythm is due to this, beta-blockers with, possibly, potassium supplements would be suitable therapy. Otherwise treatment is as for paroxysmal supraventricular tachycardia without block.

Atrial flutter

This arrhythmia seldom occurs in healthy hearts. There is usually some underlying pathology such as ischaemic or rheumatic heart disease. The ECG is characterized by coarse atrial waves (F waves) which occur with a frequency of about 300/min. They characteristically give a saw tooth apperance to the ECG usually in lead V_1 or lead II (*Fig.* 9.6).

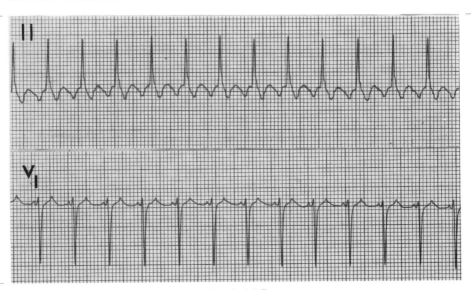

Fig. 9.6.   Atrial flutter.

There may be 1, 2, 3 or 4 F waves to each QRS complex depending on the degree of block. If, for example, there was persistent 2 F waves to 1 QRS there would be a regular, rapid heart rate.

Frequently the block varies from 3:1 to 2:1 to 4:1, etc. so that the rhythm is completely irregular and at the wrist resembles atrial fibrillation. The pressure equivalent of the coarse F waves can sometimes be seen in the neck veins.

Treatment of the underlying disorder, e.g. heart failure, often resolves the dysrhythmia. Digoxin is still the drug of choice and since it is often used also to treat the underlying cause it is most appropriate. Quinidine may also be used as may disopyramide. Cardioversion is usually successful but beta-blocking agents and verapamil are not. It is thus important to differentiate atrial flutter from paroxysmal supraventricular tachycardia if verapamil is to be used correctly. This is not always easy to do. Amiodarone is used frequently.

Atrial fibrillation

This is a very common arrhythmia and, like atrial flutter, usually is associated with underlying heart disease. There are some people – 'lone fibrillators' – in whom the heart is essentially healthy. The atria do not contract effectively and this loss of atrial contraction can be important in patients with compromised hearts such as in aortic or mitral valve stenosis because the loss of atrial 'kick' drops the cardiac output. On the ECG this is seen as low voltage irregular deviations (f waves) occurring at a frequency of 300+/min. These f waves may be coarse and resemble F waves to such an extent that it is impossible to be sure of the arrhythmia. The rate of the f waves is more rapid but in this in-between stage the term 'flutter/fibrillation' is often used. The fibrillating atria send impulses to the A-V node in a random yet rapid fashion. The pulse is irregularly irregular and the heart rate may be much higher than that recorded at the wrist. This is known as a pulse deficit. It is of little importance except as an indication that the atrial fibrillation is not yet completely controlled. Both the rate on auscultation and the rate at the wrist ought to be recorded in all patients in atrial fibrillation (*Fig.* 9.7). An apparently slow radial pulse may result in withholding digoxin if the apex (or true cardiac) rate is not checked.

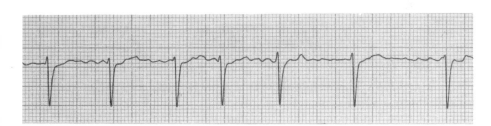

Fig. 9.7.   Atrial fibrillation.

Digoxin is the drug of choice. Beta-blocking agents may be used in addition and sometimes disopyramide is successful. If atrial fibrillation does not respond to digoxin then it is possible that the patient is thyrotoxic. Electrical cardioversion is sometimes needed and if the left atrial size is normal this should probably be attempted. Where digoxin on its own fails to control the rate verapamil, beta-blockers or amiodarone may also be used. Amiodarone may be prescribed on its own and has the added advantage of being more likely to convert the patient back to sinus rhythm. However, it has a high side-effect profile and is a potentially toxic drug in many patients.

Some patients fibrillate at a slow rate and require no active treatment except for cardioversion where appropriate.

Pre-excitation syndromes
The only common condition associated with pre-excitation is the Wolff–Parkinson–White syndrome (WPW syndrome). Pre-excitation basically means that the electrical impulse is arriving from the atria to the ventricles

earlier than would normally be expected. Thus the PR interval is short and the QRS is rather broad and has a slurred upstroke. The mechanism is due to the presence of a tract of conducting tissue which bypasses the A-V node, with its delay mechanism, and therefore allows rapid transmission of impulses from atria to ventricles. It is the electrical activity of these so-called bypass tracts that is seen as the slurred upstroke, or delta wave, on the ECG. Different destinations for the bypass tracts (right or left ventricle) have been described depending on the ECG appearances in lead V_1. If the delta wave is upright in this lead then the destination of the bypass is the right ventricle (type A WPW) (*Fig.* 9.8). Negative delta waves in lead V_1 mean a left-sided bypass tract (type B WPW). The difference is academic.

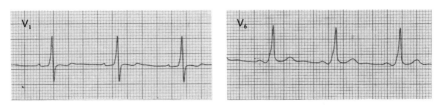

Fig. 9.8.   WPW syndrome. Leads V_1 and V_6.

The WPW syndrome predisposes to atrial tachyarrhythmias but this is not true in all cases. WPW is often seen as an incidental finding in otherwise healthy people. (Up to 1 per cent of the population may have WPW syndrome.)

The danger occurs if the bypass tract can conduct rapidly. It is not difficult to imagine the havoc that atrial fibrillation could evoke if the bypass tract conducted all f waves down to the ventricles. In patients with the WPW syndrome who are symptomatic or in high-risk employment (e.g. pilots) it is important to determine the rate at which impulses can be transmitted from atria to ventricles. In some cases this is 300+/min and such individuals are clearly at risk. Treatment is with disopyramide or amiodarone or ablation of the tract.

Ventricular ectopic beats

Ectopic beats arising from the ventricles are very common and increase in frequency with increasing age. The great majority are benign. They arise from an ectopic focus in the ventricle and are seen as broad bizarre complexes on the ECG (*Fig.* 9.9). They are commonly associated with slow heart rates and it is a useful test to see if they disappear with exercise. If they do then they are highly likely to be benign but if they increase in frequency with exercise then it is likely they represent underlying heart disease. Usually they are unifocal in which case all the ectopic complexes have the same shape and configuration. If there are two or more distinct electrocardiographic forms to the ectopic beats then they are described as multifocal and are more likely to represent underlying cardiac pathology (*Fig.* 9.10).

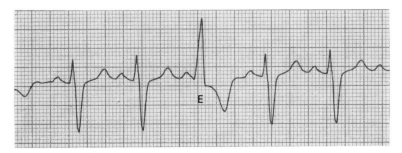

Fig. 9.9. Ventricular ectopic beat (E).

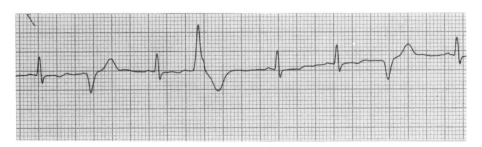

Fig. 9.10. Multifocal ventricular ectopic beats.

Ventricular ectopic beats occur early, i.e. they are seen to follow a normal QRS complex before the time of the next expected normal QRS. Following the ectopic beat there is a 'compensatory' pause so that the time interval 'normal–ectopic–normal' would be the same as 'normal–normal–normal' in time.

The patient who is aware of ectopic beats usually describes the heart as stopping and then restarting with a thump. This is really a reflection of the blood presure changes that accompany ectopic beats. As these occur early diastole is shortened, cardiac filling is shortened and the stroke volume reduced so that the patient thinks the heart has missed a beat. Conversely, with the compensatory pause diastole is lengthened, cardiac filling is increased and stroke volume is also increased. The patient feels this as a thump in the chest. Thus, frequent ectopic beats can give rise to an irregular thumping feeling in the chest (*Fig.* 9.11). As this tends to occur when the subject is settling in a chair the whole sensation can be quite alarming. It is not often that benign ventricular ectopic beats require treatment but if they do then disopyramide, mexiletine, propafenone or amiodarone are among the many drugs available. When the ectopic beats are

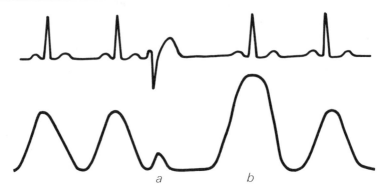

Fig. 9.11.   Effect of ventricular ectopic beats on blood pressure. At (a) the patient feels the heart 'stop' and at (b) it 'restarts' with a thump. These sensations are due to the small and large stroke volumes respectively.

not benign then the underlying heart disease should be treated although specific therapy for the ectopics may also be needed.

When the ectopic beat occurs very early then it may arrive at a time when the cardiac muscle is just recovering from a normal QRS and is electrically unstable. This is known as the 'R on T phenomenon' as the ectopic beat occurs at the time of the T wave of the preceding QRS complex. Ectopic beats at this time tend to lead to more serious rhythm disorders such as ventricular tachycardia or ventricular fibrillation. R on T ectopics are a case for specific drug treatment.

Ectopic beats may alternate with normal ones. This can give the false clinical impression of bradycardia and is known as coupling or bigeminy (*Fig.* 9.12). This too may need more active therapy.

In some patients ventricular ectopic beats may be seen to occur late rather than early. Following a normal QRS there is a pause and the expected

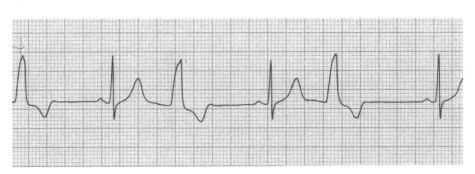

Fig. 9.12.   Ventricular bigeminy.

QRS fails to appear but soon after there is an apparent ectopic beat. This is an escape beat and means that the ventricle has spontaneously had a beat when it has not been stimulated from a higher pacing centre. These escape beats are helpful and due to the ventricle's own inherent electrical pacemaker potential. They are beneficial to the patient by aborting potential gaps in his cardiac rhythm and should not be treated.

Parasystole

Some ectopic foci discharge steadily over a longer period and on the ECG it can be seen that this regular ectopic rhythm is superimposed on the normal rhythm. Usually a long rhythm strip of ECG is needed to identify parasystole. From time to time the normal and ectopic beats will occur together (fusion beats) or one will arrive just before the other and therefore the second of the two will be inhibited. Parasystole occurs in association with organic heart disease.

Ventricular tachycardia

When three or more ectopic beats occur in rapid sequence this is known as ventricular tachycardia (*Fig.* 9.13). This is a potentially dangerous arrhythmia as the cardiac output may fall in consequence. Usually, of course, three or four

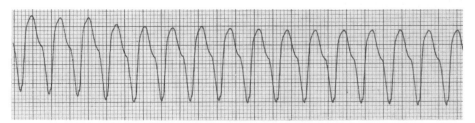

Fig. 9.13. Ventricular tachycardia.

such beats pass unnoticed but if the arrhythmia is more sustained then it can be haemodynamically very important. Ventricular tachycardia is seen in about 50 per cent of patients admitted to a coronary care unit within 24 hours. It is usually of short duration and is left untreated, but if it becomes more persistent or occurs frequently then intravenous lignocaine is used. An initial bolus of 1–2 mg/kg is given and then 1–4 mg/min. The drug is usually tailed off fairly quickly within a day or so. In severely ill patients DC shock can be used to restore the rhythm to normal but here again lignocaine can be used as maintenance therapy. Lignocaine is ineffective orally and for this reason some people prefer to use mexilitene or disopyramide, both of which are active intravenously and orally. New analogues of lignocaine are becoming available, such as tocainide, and these are also active both orally and intravenously. Amiodarone has the great advantage that it has little effect on myocardial contractility. All the other agents tend to depress cardiac function. It is given by infusion but is not as effective as it can be when in long-term use – i.e. acutely it is less anti-arrhythmic than it is after prolonged use.

Ventricular tachycardia usually represents serious underlying disease such as myocardial infarction or cardiomyopathy. It may arise from an ectopic focus (or several foci if multifocal), or be due to a re-entry mechanism. Regardless of the pathophysiology the treatment is the same for both. Long-term therapy is with disopyramide, mexilitene or amiodarone or sometimes a combination. The beta-blocker sotalol has some amiodarone-like activity and can be used.

Ventricular fibrillation

This is one form of cardiac arrest and is characterized by rapid ineffective twitching of the ventricular muscle. This is paralleled by rapid bizarre small voltage complexes on the ECG (*Fig.* 9.14). It occurs most commonly in patients with myocardial infarction. There seem to be two types of patients affected: one

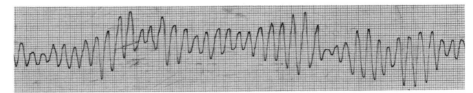

Fig. 9.14.   Ventricular fibrillation.

with recent infarction who develops ventricular fibrillation, is successfully treated, and in whom the heart is basically sound. The prognosis here is good. The other is when ventricular fibrillation is almost an agonal rhythm in patients who have cardiogenic shock or heart failure. Often these patients can be resuscitated but their prognosis even in the short term is poor.

Treatment is with DC shock and maintenance therapy is as for ventricular tachycardia. Most physicians would continue with oral therapy for several months in the low-risk group and indefinitely in the high-risk group.

● Bradyarrhythmias

Sinus bradycardia

There is some dispute as to whether sinus bradycardia is defined as a heart rate of less than 60 beats/min or less than 50 beats/min. It is probably best defined as an inappropriately slow pulse rate for the patient's age and circumstances and should be decided on an individual basis. A slow heart rate may reflect sino-atrial disease especially in an older person. Beta-blocking agents slow the heart rate, sometimes markedly, and drug ingestion should be asked about in the history.

Sinus arrest

Whole complexes may be missing from the ECG and there may be fairly long pauses in the cardiac rhythm often terminated by an escape beat. As with sinus bradycardia this may occur in normal people with high vagal tone but is more usually a reflection of an abnormal sino-atrial node.

Sino-atrial block

The sinus node generates an electrical signal but this is not conducted to the atria. On the ECG QRS complexes are missing but in multiples of the normal R-R interval. Thus if one QRS complex is blocked in sino-atrial (exit) block the next QRS complex after that will arrive on time. This abnormality usually reflects sinus node disease.

Tachycardia-bradycardia syndrome

This syndrome is being recognized increasingly especially with the more widespread use of 24-hour ECG monitoring. It is also known as the sick sinus syndrome or abbreviated to the tachy-brady syndrome. Sick sinus syndrome is a useful description as it reflects sino-atrial disease. There are episodes of tachycardia such as atrial fibrillation or supraventricular tachycardia together with episodes of bradycardia such as sinus arrest or heart block. These abnormalities tend to be intermittent. Drug therapy can be unsatisfactory because any drug slowing the heart rate (such as digoxin or beta-blockers) and being used to treat the tachyarrhythmias will make the bradyarrhythmia worse. Often drugs and an endocardial pacemaker have to be used together.

In some patients intracardiac electrocardiography may need to be performed to detect the abnormality in sinus node function, e.g. prolonged sinus node recovery time. In addition there is often disease in other parts of the conduction system which can be detected at the same time.

If a patient with the sick sinus syndrome is suffering only palpitations then a drug like disopyramide can be used. There is little evidence that pacemaker insertions prophylactically in such patients are helpful as the outlook is good in any case. In the patient who is having syncopal episodes associated with bradyarrhythmias a pacemaker should be inserted.

Heart block

This is a relatively common disorder, has varying degrees of severity, and is usually a result of idiopathic fibrosis or degeneration of the conducting system. Less often ischaemic heart disease is the cause and other rarer aetiologies include drugs such as digoxin and beta-blocking agents. The calcification associated with aortic stenosis may extend into the conducting tissue and cause heart block. In these patients it is important to know whether their syncopal episodes are effort related and whether their 12-lead (or ambulatory 24-hour) ECG shows any evidence of conduction disturbance.

First-degree AV Block

This is entirely free of symptoms but shows up on the ECG as a prolonged PR interval (the time from the onset of the P wave to the onset of the QRS complex). The PR interval ought to be less than 0.20–0.21 s. The PR interval can be so long that the P wave is almost superimposed on the preceding T wave (*Fig. 9.15*). A prolonged PR interval is not always pathological as it can be seen in people with a high vagal tone (e.g. young athletes).

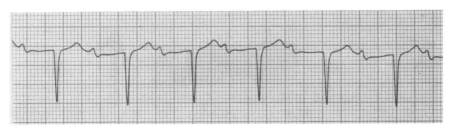

Fig. 9.15.   First-degree heart block.

Second-degree AV block

The terminology of second-degree AV block is confusing largely because two synonymous terms have been used to decribe the same electrocardiographic appearance. Mobitz type I is also known as Wenckebach phenomenon. Here the PR interval lengthens with each succeeding beat until finally an atrial complex (P wave) is not followed by a QRS complex. A dropped beat therefore occurs (*Fig. 9.16*).

Mobitz type II AV block occurs when not all atrial complexes are conducted to the ventricles but those that are have a consistent, unvarying PR interval. The

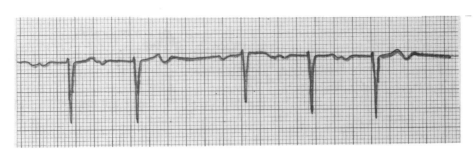

Fig. 9.16.   Mobitz type I – Wenckebach.

degree of block, i.e. 2:1, 3:1, etc., can vary but the PR interval does not (*Fig. 9.17*). This is generally regarded as a more serious arrhythmia than Mobitz type I.

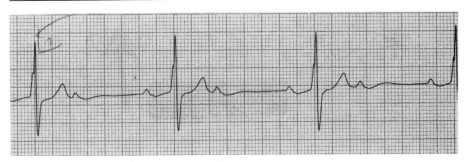

Fig. 9.17. Mobitz type II.

Third-degree AV block (complete heart block)

Here there is complete dissociation between P waves and QRS complexes (*Fig. 9.18*). The P waves are usually more frequent and atrial activity is not conducted to the ventricles. The ventricular rate can be very slow indeed and can be punctuated by pauses or asystole (Stokes–Adams attacks). Such pauses are usually symptomatic and require urgent hospital admission. Where the rate is relatively slow but stable the patient may develop heart failure as a result.

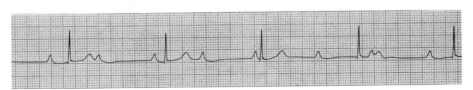

Fig. 9.18. Complete heart block.

Treatment

First-degree heart block and Wenckebach phenomenon (Mobitz type I) do not require treatment although the patients may be aware of the dropped beat with the latter. Mobitz type II and third-degree heart block usually require insertion of a permanent pacemaker system.

10

Heart failure

Heart failure may predominantly affect the left heart, the right heart or both. It may be acute or chronic. The patient admitted as an emergency will be in acute left ventricular failure. Although successfully treated he may end up with chronic left ventricular failure and right ventricular failure (congestive cardiac failure).

The causes of left ventricular failure are:
1. Volume overload e.g. Mitral incompetence
                          Aortic incompetence
2. Pressure overload e.g. Aortic stenosis
                          Systemic hypertension
3. Myocardial failure e.g. Coronary artery disease
                           Cardiomyopathy
4. Arrhythmias which may produce left ventricular failure *per se* or as a complication of any of the above.
5. Drugs.
6. Secondary to systemic disease, e.g. myxoedema, anaemia.

Mitral stenosis causes pulmonary oedema as does left ventricular failure (LVF) and their treatment is the same. Note that although mitral stenosis causes pulmonary oedema it is not due to LVF. The treatment of heart failure in any form is divided into:
1. Symptomatic treatment of the heart failure itself.
2. The treatment of the underlying cause.

● **Treatment of acute left ventricular failure (LVF)**
1. Sit the patient up and administer 100 per cent oxygen. Sitting the patient upright reduces the venous return to the heart and reduces the preload. In moderate left ventricular failure the PO_2 may be 5–6 kPa and 100 per cent oxygen will rapidly improve this towards normal.

154

2.   Intravenous diuretic.
      Preload will be reduced markedly by a diuretic but diuretics cause a fluid shift out of the perialveolar spaces within minutes of administration. Whatever the cause of heart failure an intravenous diuretic should be given first (e.g. frusemide 80 mg, bumetanide 2 mg).
3.   Digoxin.
      Digoxin has a positive inotropic action without increasing the oxygen demand. It is thus of great value in cardiac failure but it has its drawbacks. Given orally its onset of action is slow (several hours) but intravenously it must be administered carefully or dangerous arrhythmias may occur and its total effect is still not immediate. Digoxin 0.25 mg in 50 ml dextrose (5 per cent) given over 30 minutes is quite safe. Even so, its action is by no means as rapid as a diuretic.
4.   Treatment of arrhythmias.
      If the precipitating cause of left ventricular failure is an arrhythmia it must be dealt with rapidly either by DC shock or intravenous anti-arrhythmics (see chapter 9). Occasionally the arrhythmia may be digoxin induced or may be made worse by digoxin.
5.   Opiates.
      Intravenous morphine reduces left ventricular end diastolic pressure and pulmonary artery pressure. It also sedates the patient and removes the usually substantial anxiety and distress that accompanies LVF. There is also, probably, a mild diuretic effect.
6.   Aminophylline.
      The indication for this drug is less clear but it is still widely used. It is a bronchodilator but also has positive inotropic and chronotropic effects on the heart. Given too rapidly it may produce dangerous arrhythmias or even cardiac arrest.
7.   Vasodilators.
      Occasionally left ventricular failure cannot be relieved by digoxin and diuretics alone. By reducing the afterload with a vasodilator the left ventricle will be able to increase its stroke volume and therefore cardiac output also rises (*Fig.* 10.1).
      The drugs which are commonly used are:
   a.   Sodium nitroprusside (reduces preload) intravenous only
   b.   Hydralazine (reduces afterload)
   c.   Glyceryl trinitrate or other nitrates (mainly reduces preload)
   d.   Prazosin (reduces preload and afterload)
      These drugs can be used intravenously but may precipitously drop the blood pressure. Oral therapy is, therefore, better but the blood pressure must still be carefully monitored. Preload- and afterload-reducing agents may be used simultaneously.
8.   Venesection.
   a.   Surgical
         Removal of a pint of blood by placing a needle in an antecubital vein may

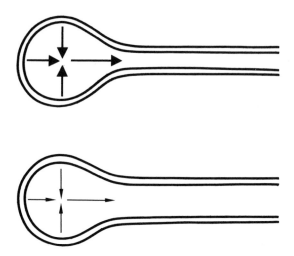

Fig. 10.1. Effect of vasodilator on myocardial work. Peripheral resistance is reduced, therefore the heart meets with less obstruction to its ejection and work is therefore reduced while cardiac output rises.

be life saving when all else fails. It reduces the preload extremely rapidly and it can be repeated once.

b. Medical
Tourniquets round the lower limbs blown up to about 50 mmHg will prevent venous return from these areas to the heart and thus reduce preload. The cuffs must be deflated for 30 minutes every hour and the benefit is therefore only temporary.

● **Treatment of chronic left ventricular failure**

1. Mild
Many patients will lead a normal life taking oral diuretics and digoxin. A usual regimen would be:
Digoxin 0.25 mg
Thiazide diuretic or loop diuretic – one tablet daily together with potassium supplements or potassium-sparing diuretic (often combined in the same tablet).

2. Moderate
These patients may need a larger dose of diuretic in addition to their digoxin. If this is not controlling the failure, oral vasodilators can be introduced, e.g. angiotensin converting enzyme (ACE) inhibitors.

3.   Severe
      Digoxin, diuretics and vasodilators must be used and if these are not
      controlling the symptoms consider:
  a. Reducing sodium intake.
  b. Daily period of rest in bed.
  c. Fluid restriction.
      It is extremely important at the onset of left ventricular failure that a
cause be sought and treated if possible.

● **Treatment of the causes of left ventricular failure**
1.   Volume overload
      Prosthetic valve replacement.
2.   Pressure overload
      Prosthetic valve replacement for aortic stenosis and adequate therapy for
      systemic hypertension.
3.   Myocardial failure
      Reducing risk factors (smoking, hypertension) may prevent worsening of
      coronary artery disease but there is little evidence yet that coronary
      artery bypass grafting will generally improve left ventricular function,
      although it may do in individual cases. Removal of a left ventricular
      aneurysm may, however, be successful. Left ventricular failure may be
      precipitated by a myocardial infarction so that serial ECGs and enzyme
      estimations may be necessary. If there is a cause for a cardiomyopathy
      (e.g. alcohol) some improvement of function may be obtained by
      removing it.
4.   Arrhythmias
      Appropriate drug treatment.
5.   Systemic disease
      Treatment of myxoedema or anaemia, etc. as appropriate.
6.   Drugs
      Stop any offending drug if at all possible, e.g. beta-blocking agents.

● **Treatment of right ventricular failure**
      Most cases of right ventricular failure are secondary to left ventricular
failure. Treatment of the latter therefore treats the former. Right ventricular
failure on its own is treated along similar lines to left ventricular failure and the
underlying causes should be dealt with appropriately.
1.   Volume overload
      Pulmonary incompetence.
      Tricuspid incompetence.
      Surgical intervention if absolutely essential. Surgery to these valves is not
      ideal and not always necessary or successful.

2.   Pressure overload
      Pulmonary stenosis – treat surgically as this is very successful (or by balloon valvuloplasty).
      Pulmonary hypertension – treat cause if possible, but no drugs have been shown to be generally effective in reducing the pulmonary artery pressure. However, nifedipine, ACE inhibitors and nitrates may benefit individual patients.
3.   Myocardial failure. ⎫
4.   Arrhythmias.   ⎪
5.   Drugs.   ⎬ As for left ventricular failure
6.   Systemic disease.   ⎭

● **Important points**

Digoxin
      It is doubtful, despite its benefits, whether digoxin would be allowed on to the market if it was discovered today because of the very narrow margin between therapeutic and toxic doses. The physiological effects on the heart are:
  a. Increase in the force and velocity of contraction (useful in heart failure).
  b. Decreases impulse conduction in the atrioventricular (AV) node (useful for tachyarrhythmias but not for the WPW syndrome where it is contraindicated).
  c. Increases automaticity of secondary pacemakers (results in arrhythmias if there is digoxin toxicity).
      Toxicity occurs in 8 per cent of patients on digoxin alone and up to 24 per cent in those also on a diuretic. Toxicity is more likely if:
  a. Potassium falls below 3.5 mmol/l or exceeds 5 mmol/l. Because most patients are also on a diuretic potassium variations can be considerable.
  b. Renal function is impaired. Digoxin is 80 per cent excreted by the kidneys.
  c. The patient is elderly. Excretion is reduced.
      Toxic effects are:
  a. Gastrointestinal upsets. Anorexia, nausea and occasionally diarrhoea.
  b. Arrhythmias. Every arrhythmia can occur with digoxin but a sinus bradycardia, ventricular ectopics, particularly bigeminal rhythm and paroxysmal atrial tachycardia with varying block, are the arrhythmias typically associated with the drug.
      Rarely xanthopsia (yellow vision) may occur. Because digoxin is so liable to toxicity the indications for its use must be precise. They are:
  a. Acute left ventricular failure with sinus rhythm or atrial fibrillation.
  b. Tachyarrhythmias. Atrial fibrillation or flutter with rapid ventricular rate. Supraventricular tachycardia (but not WPW syndrome).

c.   Maintenance therapy in chronic left ventricular failure (although widely used there is still some doubt whether this is beneficial to patients in sinus rhythm).

Serum digoxin levels can be estimated. This is very valuable in cases where toxicity is suspected or where an arrhythmia is not responding to treatment by digoxin and it is not known whether the patient is receiving too much or too little. The normal range is 1.5–3.0 μg/l (pg/ml) – 8 hours after the last dose. More recently these levels have been found to be elevated when the digoxin dosage remains unchanged but the patient is also given nifedipine, verapamil or amiodarone.

Digitalization of a patient must be performed very carefully. Normal oral digitalization (Lanoxin) varies according to the patient but possible regimens are as follows:

Normal adult patient   0.25 mg three times daily for day 1 (orally)
0.25 mg twice daily for day 2
0.25 mg daily thereafter.

A patient in whom toxicity is likely (variable K^+, renal function, old age), 0.25 mg twice daily for day 1 (orally), 0.625 mg daily thereafter.

There is great variation in the way patients are digitalized and no one method is correct.

Digoxin toxicity may be treated in the following ways:

a.   Stopping the digoxin.
b.   Correcting potassium levels as appropriate.
c.   If tachyarrhythmias are present a beta-blocking agent is the drug of choice either intravenously or orally.
d.   If atrioventricular block is present a temporary pacemaker may be necessary.
e.   If a tachyarrhythmia is present more urgent treatment may occasionally be necessary and cardioversion with a DC shock may be essential. This must be performed with intravenous beta-blocker cover and a pacemaker *in situ*. Cardioversion should begin at 5 J and be slowly increased. With a digitalized patient cardioversion carries a high risk of asystole or other serious dysrhythmia.

Diuretics

Thiazides act in the ascending limb of the loop of Henle preventing sodium reabsorption and interfering with dilution. Frusemide and bumetanide act in the loop of Henle and its ascending limb, having a more potent action than thiazides. Aldosterone antagonists prevent potassium excretion and increase sodium excretion in the distal convoluted tubule. A combination of thiazides and frusemide or bumetanide can be additive because they do not work in the same way. A combination of frusemide or bumetanide plus an aldosterone antagonist is very useful because they, too, work in different ways.

Diuretics have side effects. Hypovolaemia is common with a rise in blood urea. This can easily cause confusion in the elderly. Thiazides can precipitate both gout and hyperglycaemia in susceptible patients. Thiazides, frusemide and bumetanide can cause profound potassium depletion and patients usually require potassium supplements or potassium-sparing diuretics in addition. (These diuretics seem to cause more potassium loss in heart failure than is normally seen when they are used to treat high blood pressure.) If a combination of such diuretics is used (e.g. frusemide and spironolactone) where one drug causes potassium loss and the other conserves it, supplementary potassium may be dangerous.

ACE inhibitors

These drugs, e.g. captopril, enalapril, lisinopril cause a reduction of both angiotensin II and aldosterone. The effect of the former is to result in vasodilatation while the reduction in aldosterone reduces sodium and hence water retention. These are valuable assets in treating heart failure but the drop in blood pressure they cause may be too great to be tolerated. There is, however, a move to introduce ACE inhibitors earlier and earlier in the management of heart failure. They have been shown to improve both the quality and quantity of these patients' lives.

11

Hypertension

High blood pressure has proved over the years to be very hard to define. It is known that in western countries at least, the blood pressure increases with age so that what might be regarded as a high pressure level in a 20-year-old would be perfectly acceptable in his grandparents. Arterial blood pressure is also normally distributed in the population (*Fig.* 11.1) with only a slight skewing to the right to account for secondary hypertension. Therefore some people have 'high' pressure compared with the average, but the point at which this term would be used is purely arbitrary.

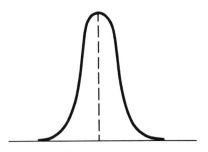

Fig. 11.1.   Normal distribution curve.

If a patient was to walk into his family doctor's office and have his blood pressure checked a dozen times over the next half hour it is doubtful whether the same reading would be obtained twice. The blood pressure is extremely variable from minute to minute and of particular importance in determining a patient's blood pressure is to recognize the effect that alerting or defence reactions can have on the level obtained. In the course of a normal day the blood pressure may vary in value by as much as 100 per cent or more. In particular the level is often very low during sleep (diastolic levels of 40 or 50 mmHg are not uncommon) and extremely high during exercise or sexual intercourse. Systolic blood pressures of more than 300 mmHg have been recorded in people stepping out of sauna baths straight into the icy sea.

Fig. 11.2 shows a typical intra-arterial 24-hour blood pressure trace from a subject wearing portable recording apparatus and in whom there was an indwelling cannula in the brachial artery.

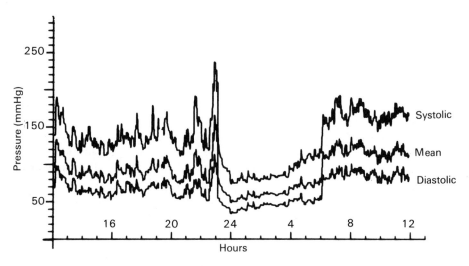

Fig. 11.2. Twenty-four-hour blood pressure record showing systolic, mean and diastolic pressures.

Taking all these considerations into account we do know, however, that when a subject walks into the outpatient clinic, surgery or office and has his blood pressure measured the reading obtained has predictive value for that individual's future. If the pressure is high on such an occasion it is likely that the individual has or will develop sustained hypertension. Unfortunately this is not invariable as there is a considerable percentage of people in whom subsequent blood pressure measurements will reveal the pressure to be normal. In general, though, even the roughest of blood pressure measurements tends not to be too far from the long-term truth.

Children with higher than average blood pressures tend to grow into adults with higher than average pressures. The same holds true for those with lower pressures. Thus it may be possible to detect the population at risk at a very early stage. Naturally one would be reluctant to start school children on therapy for high blood pressure but a routine school blood pressure measurement might prove a good way to screen the population and to identify those people likely to be at risk later in life.

● Blood pressure measurement

The technique of blood pressure measurement is all important. Far too often the person measuring the blood pressure has had no formal teaching in how to do it and does not appreciate the pitfalls. The cuff should be applied to the arm with the rubber balloon over the artery. For the average person the cuff should be 13 cm wide but large cuffs are needed for fat arms and in thin people or children smaller cuff sizes are used. The radial pulse should be palpated at the wrist as the cuff is inflated fairly rapidly. In this way the observer has an idea of the systolic pressure. Next inflate the cuff another 20–30 mmHg above the level at which the radial pulse disappeared. Now place the stethoscope diaphragm over the brachial artery and let down the sphygmomanometer pressure slowly at 2 mmHg/s, listening all the while for the Korotkoff sounds.

Korotkoff sounds

There are five different sounds heard at various stages as the cuff pressure is released. The first Korotkoff sound is the initial beat that is heard and this is the systolic pressure. Next, this sound becomes muffled (phase II) or may even disappear. The pitfall here is obvious and is the reason for palpating the systolic pressure at the wrist as the cuff is inflated. Phase III is where the sounds become louder and harsher once more, or if the sounds disappeared at phase II they reappear at phase III. Phase IV occurs when the sounds once more become muffled and phase V is where they finally disappear. In some patients there is no phase V and Korotkoff sounds can still be heard when the sphygmomanometer is recording 0 mmHg. The reason for this is not known but it is seen sometimes in normals; more commonly it is seen in some medical conditions such as anaemia and in particular in patients with aortic valve incompetence. In drug studies phase IV tends to be taken as the diastolic pressure but when phase IV is compared directly with arterial recordings performed from a cannula in the other brachial artery, this phase consistently is about 5 mmHg or so higher than true diastole. Phase V which probably is used by most clinicians and nurses is more readily definable in the vast majority of subjects but compared with direct arterial pressure recordings tends to underestimate the diastolic pressure by 4–5 mmHg (see *Fig.* 3.8).

The World Health Organization suggests that a blood pressure of 160/95 or above is abnormal. For practical purposes this level, confirmed on several clinic visits, is probably a good dividing point at least up to the age of 60 or so. A higher pressure might be allowable in an older person although evidence that the pressure is causing target organ damage in any patient would make it more likely that treatment should be started.

● Presentation

Patients who have high blood pressure are generally completely symptom-free and well. The elevated pressure is a risk factor for cardiovascular damage and is not usually thought of as a disease as such. The end points are of course disastrous with myocardial infarcts or cerebrovascular accidents being by far the commonest. High blood pressure prematurely ages the circulation so that these disasters occur at a much earlier age than would otherwise be expected. It is difficult to persuade any one individual that he or she is at risk. People do not believe that 'it will happen to them' and compliance is often a problem. It is essential from this point of view that any therapy started does not render a well individual unwell.

It is reckoned that about 10 per cent of the populations of the United Kingdom (5 000 000 people) and the United States (20 000 000) have elevated blood pressures to such an extent that they are at risk. Of these about 50 per cent are undetected (12 500 000); 25 per cent are not on therapy even though high blood pressure has been detected (6 250 000) and 12.5 per cent are on treatment but blood pressure is inadequately controlled (3 125 000). This leaves one-eighth properly managed. Clearly there is a need for education of both public and medical profession alike.

In the UK 90 per cent of a general practitioner's patients will visit him within a 3-year period. If the doctor were to measure all his patient's blood pressures just once in this period then virtually everyone in the country with an elevated blood pressure would be found.

● Cause of high blood pressure

In the vast majority of people no cause can be found for their high blood pressure. These people are considered to have 'primary' or 'essential' hypertension and constitute more than 95 per cent of the total. They often have a family history of hypertension and there is a great deal of epidemiological evidence showing the trends in high blood pressure in their near relatives. All the different mechanisms in the body that control blood pressure have been implicated at some time in the aetiology of essential hypertension. These include the renin–angiotensin system, the baroreceptors, the sympathetic nervous system, the kidney and salt excretion, primary structural changes in the blood vessels and a variety of others. It is unlikely, however, that there is a single cause for high blood pressure and it may well require interplay of several factors, e.g. environment and genetic predisposition, etc.

● Secondary hypertension

In a few patients a cause can be found for their elevated pressure. These account for less than 5 per cent of the total and in only a few is there specific therapy different from that adopted for essential hypertension. For these reasons there has been a considerable move away from investigating hypertension clinically in any great depth unless there are highly specific indications from the history, or examination, or where the patient is young (under 35–40 years) when the percentage of secondary hypertension is considerably higher.

Causes of secondary hypertension
1.   Endocrine
2.   Renal
3.   Coarctation of aorta
4.   Pregnancy

1.   *Endocrine*

Contraceptive pill
In most women oral contraceptives will cause the blood pressure to rise by a few mmHg. This is usually of little consequence and the blood pressure reverts to previous levels when the contraceptive agent is stopped. Pre-existing hypertension is a relative contraindication to prescribing oral contraceptives. In a very small number of females the pill results in more severe hypertension and there have been a few cases of malignant phase hypertension reported.

Cushing's syndrome
There is hyperplasia of the adrenal gland and over-production of steroid hormones. This is a condition that is more likely to come to the attention of the endocrinologist but an elevated blood pressure is part of the clinical picture.

Steroid therapy itself can cause an elevation of blood pressure when used in long-term management of such conditions as asthma, the lymphomas or rheumatoid arthritis. Usually these preparations are given for very good reasons and cannot be stopped.

Conn's syndrome
This is a rare condition characterized by a low serum potassium level. The vast majority of hypertensive people in whom the serum potassium is low do not have Conn's syndrome. For instance most of the thiazide diuretics can cause hypokalaemia to varying degrees.

The pressure elevation is due to over-production of the potent mineralocorticoid aldosterone. Conn's syndrome is also known as primary aldosteronism. While some cases are due to adrenal tumours many are due to nodular hyperplasia of the glands. In either case management is largely medical with the aldosterone antagonist, spironolactone, which can be dramatically effective when difficulty in blood pressure control has been a problem with other drugs.

The clinical picture is of weakness, headache and thirst all of which are rather non-specific. Diagnosis can be confirmed by measuring the plasma aldosterone levels.

Phaeochromocytomas
These tumours may be malignant although most are benign and they are usually found in the adrenal gland but may occur elsewhere, e.g. in the paravertebral groove, in other parts of the abdomen or rarely in the bladder. The tumours secrete catecholamines, either noradenaline or adrenaline, and this secretion is

usually sustained but may be sporadic. This is reflected in the blood pressure which is more usually persistently elevated rather than intermittently raised.

Phaeochromocytomas are not uncommon, being found at post mortem in 1 per cent of hypertensive patients. They are diagnosed much less frequently during life. These tumours should be suspected in someone with rapidly increasing blood pressure or with hypertension of short duration. Similarly they should be sought in patients with very variable levels of hypertension. All young people (less than 40) should be screened if their blood pressure is elevated.

Presentation may simply be with high blood pressure but an associated history of flushing, palpitations, headaches and weight loss ought to alert the doctor to the possibility of a phaeochromocytoma. There may also be episodes of sudden unexplained pallor. The blood pressure is said not to fall at night in patients with these tumours.

Screening of patients is by checking the urinary vanillyl mandelic acid in 24-hour urine samples. It ought to be raised, but is relatively insensitive and tumours may be missed. More specific are the urinary metanephrines and normetanephrines, metabolites of adrenaline and noradrenaline respectively. Plasma catecholamines are increasingly being measured directly.

The tumour is seldom identifiable on clinical examination although rarely an abdominal mass can be palpated. In such cases handling of the tumour can lead to release of catecholamines into the blood stream and massive rises in blood pressure. Great care must therefore be taken in examining someone with a suspected phaeochromocytoma and direct handling kept to the absolute minimum.

Arteriography is usually required to locate the tumour (or tumours – they can be multiple). This should only be done by people experienced in dealing with phaeochromocytomas and only after the patient has been fully adrenergically blocked, first of all with alpha-blocking agents (usually phenoxybenzamine) and then beta-blocking agents (e.g. atenolol). Some physicians use the combined alpha- and beta-blocking agent labetalol.

At surgery the tumour can be removed but, again, handling should be kept to the absolute minimum. An interesting transition occurs during surgery in that the patient, who is fully alpha- and beta-blocked to resist the catecholamines from the tumour, suddenly becomes completely over-treated when the tumour is removed. Catecholamines may even need to be infused to keep up the blood pressure. It is obvious that an experienced team is required to handle the surgical management of these tumours.

2.   *Renal causes*
Virtually any renal disease can cause high blood pressure. It is even seen in renal transplant patients although they may, of course, be on steroid therapy as well.
   Renal artery stenosis
This should be suspected with relatively recent onset of hypertension and especially if it appears to be accelerated. A bruit may be heard over the offending kidney or in the epigastrium but as often as not there are no physical

signs. The artery is usually stenosed by atheroma but fibromuscular dysplasia is also a common cause in younger patients.

The intravenous pyelogram (IVP) shows delayed excretion of dye in the affected kidney, which is smaller than normal. Later films will show that the dye on the affected side is slower to clear so that there appears to be a greater concentration of dye on the affected side. All or none of these may be present in a patient with renal artery stenosis. They reflect simply the reduction in blood flow past the stenosis. Renal ultrasound may detect the smaller kidney. Selective renal arteriography is the next step to delineate the stenosis and to see if it is amenable to surgical correction. At the same time renal vein renins are usually measured and these are found to be elevated on the affected side.

Some of these lesions are amenable to balloon dilatation (angioplasty). An experienced radiologist will often go ahead and do this at the time of the angiogram if the anatomy looks suitable.

Surgical reconstruction of the artery (either endarterectomy or bypass grafting) results in cure in about 50 per cent of these patients while blood pressure levels will be substantially reduced in another 35 per cent.

Pyelonephritis

This has to be long standing before the blood pressure is affected. Even in cases where the IVP suggests predominantly the involvement of one kidney, it is virtually certain that both are involved. Therefore, unilateral nephrectomy has not been a great success and management is largely with drugs.

Other renal causes

Analgesic nephropathy used to be common but now that the dangers of phenacetin (causes renal papillary necrosis) are better known this is less of a problem. Renal artery emboli occasionally occur as do renin secreting tumours.

Coarctation of aorta (see chapter 7)

This is congenital narrowing of the aorta just where the ductus arteriosus connected the aorta and pulmonary artery *in utero*. Characteristically there is high blood pressure in the upper limbs and low or normal blood pressure in the legs. Often the femoral pulses can be palpated but they are delayed when simultaneously compared with the radial pulses. These children may present early in life with heart failure or later when the coarctation is an incidental finding and certainly the femoral pulses ought to be examined in every hypertensive patient.

In general the results from the point of view of future blood pressure control are better if the coarctation is corrected early. This is generally done before school age but there is some evidence that treatment even earlier would be better still. There is often associated aortic stenosis and intracranial berry aneurysms. The combination of berry aneurysm and high blood pressure is especially dangerous. The operation carries a substantial recurrence rate although newer techniques have reduced this to about 10–15 per cent in 5 years. Even those subjects with a good repair may remain hypertensive and the majority of patients require antihypertensive therapy at some stage.

4.   *Pregnancy*

Eclampsia is a condition in pregnancy where the mother is extremely ill. It is associated with very high blood pressure and great risk to both mother and fetus.

Much more common is pre-eclamptic toxaemia where the blood pressure is mildly raised, the ankles swell and there may be proteinuria. It usually responds to bed rest, sedation and, if necessary, fairly gentle antihypertensive treatment, e.g. nifedipine. Patients who have had either form of toxaemia often go on to develop high blood pressure later in life and it is something that should be asked about in the history when assessing a hypertensive patient.

No manufacturer is prepared to recommend his product for pregnant females with high blood pressure but methyldopa, propranolol, atenolol, hydralazine and labetalol have been used and are probably safe. Nifedipine is also widely used.

● **Assessment of the hypertensive patient**

The history and physical examination are by far the most important part of assessing patients with high blood pressure. In the history particular interest should be centred on any drug ingestion, including the contraceptive pill which is often not considered by the patient as a drug. Symptoms referable to any of the secondary causes of high blood pressure should be sought and also the family history determined.

Physical examination should have two objectives: to determine whether the patient does indeed have high blood pressure and also to determine its severity. Any evidence of secondary hypertension or of target organ damage is sought for.

The heart may be enlarged clinically and often the aortic component of the second sound is loud (loud A_2). The optic fundi are particularly useful in assessing the severity of hypertension. The Keith–Wagener classification is used to describe them.

0   Normal fundi

I   Arteries straighter, narrower and reflect light more than normal (silver wiring).

II   The arteries cause the veins to be compressed where they cross over each other – AV nipping.

III   Grade II + haemorrhages and exudates.

IV   Papilloedema – i.e. oedema of the optic disc and loss of its clear margins.

Grades III–IV represent severe degrees of high blood pressure and such an individual should be admitted to hospital for treatment. Grades I and II are very non-specific and are seen in normotensive people as they age. It is the premature appearance of such changes that should be considered in assessing the patient.

The kidneys should be palpated and renal artery bruits looked for, femoral arteries palpated and blood pressure determined in both arms and, where appropriate, the legs.

Every patient should have the urine dip tested, an MSU (mid-stream specimen of urine) together with blood urea and electrolytes, creatinine, haemoglobin, chest X-ray and ECG. These last two assess the degree to which the heart has become enlarged or hypertrophied in response to the elevated pressure.

In a middle-aged patient if these initial tests are all satisfactory then investigations go no further. In a younger patient (under 40 or so) then a VMA and IVP should be performed. Where appropriate further specialized tests should be carried out but this is very much the exception.

● **Pathological consequences of high blood pressure**

High blood pressure causes the cardiovascular system to wear badly and to age prematurely. If the patient smokes and is overweight the wear and tear is increased. The results of hypertension are shown in *Figs*. 11.3–11.5 and 12.4–12.6.

A.   Myocardial infarction and heart failure (*Fig*. 11.3).
B.   Cerebrovascular accident (*Fig*. 11.4).
C.   Renal failure (*Fig*. 11.5).
D.   Dissecting aneurysm (see *Figs*. 12.4–12.6).

● **Treatment**

Treatment of high blood pressure is worthwhile. Surprisingly there used to be some doubt about this but a series of studies have shown that virtually all groups of patients with elevated blood pressure will do better on treatment. There remains the very mild or labile hypertensive where treatment has yet to be of proven value. The problem here, as mentioned earlier, is to determine which of these people really are hypertensive in the first place. The elderly do seem to benefit from therapy although this was long in doubt. Myocardial infarction rates were not reduced initially with the older anti-hypertensive drugs although the other end points of hypertension were. It remains to be seen whether with the newer anti-hypertensive drugs the infarct rate also declines.

Anti-hypertensive therapy

There does at last seem to be some agreement in the general approach to high blood pressure. Obviously a few cases of secondary hypertension will have specific remedies, e.g. removal of a phaeochromocytoma, but in the vast majority of cases, including most secondary hypertensives, therapy is started

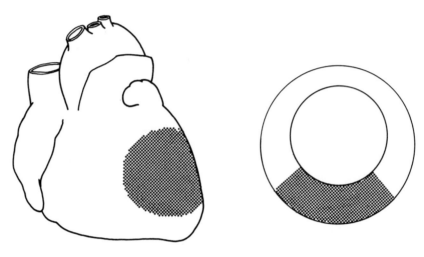

Fig. 11.3.   Myocardial infarction.

with either a diuretic agent or a beta-blocking drug. The argument has raged as to which of these two should be used first.

Diuretics and beta-adrenoceptor blocking agents are about equi-potent and effect moderate reductions in blood pressure. Diuretics seem able to potentiate the hypotensive effects of other drugs. Both types of drugs have side effects of which diuretics are arguably potentially more serious. Most physicians are in agreement, however, that if treatment is started with a beta-blocker then a diuretic should be the next choice and *vice versa* if the diuretic is used first.

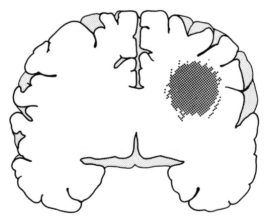

Fig. 11.4.   Cerebrovascular accident.

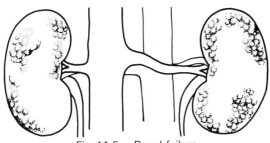

Fig. 11.5.   Renal failure.

Diuretic therapy

It is conventional to use a thiazide diuretic in the treatment of high blood pressure. Loop diuretics (such as frusemide and bumetanide) also lower blood pressure but tend to be less effective and more expensive. There are many thiazide diuretics but bendrofluazide, hydrochlorothiazide and chlorthalidone are the most widely used. Proprietary preparations such as Moduretic (amiloride, hydrochlorothiazide) and Dyazide (hydrochlorothiazide, triamterene) also contain potassium-sparing diuretics to offset the tendency to hypokalaemia with the thiazides. Hypokalaemia is not a major feature with the thiazides provided the dose is kept within the recommended maximum. Hypokalaemia tends to be dose dependent while increasing the dose does not increase the anti-hypertensive efficacy of the drugs. Diuretics also predispose to gout, diabetes and to dehydration but despite this the thiazides are, in general, safe, cheap and effective. They may cause impotence in males.

Beta-adrenoceptor blocking agents

There are now many of these available. Some have long half-lives and can be given once daily, e.g. acebutolol and atenolol; others have been advocated for once-daily use in slow-release form, e.g. oxprenolol, propranolol and metoprolol. Some are cardioselective in that they block only beta-one receptors. This makes them less likely to provoke bronchospasm in susceptible individuals. Examples of cardioselective agents are atenolol and metoprolol. Beta-blocking agents can provoke bronchospasm and they make heart failure worse or make incipient heart failure overt. Other side effects include cold hands and feet and, in rare cases, gangrene, bad dreams and impotence. In general, though, beta-blockers are safe and effective. It is probably better to use one that can be given once daily and that is cardioselective. Many physicians prefer to remain with the tried and trusted propranolol in which case the slow release form (Inderal LA) is probably the best to increase compliance.

Combined preparations of beta-blockers and diuretics

An increasing number of these preparations are appearing on the market. They make sense from the point of view of compliance and are suitable for use as a single tablet taken once daily. Used in this way they do lower the blood pressure and can be effective. The problem arises when the doctor wishes to increase the dose as then he has to increase both diuretic and beta-blocker simultaneously.

Vasodilator therapy

When beta-blockers and diuretics have been used and have failed to lower the blood pressure to acceptable levels it is now usual to add in a vasodilator agent. The ones commonly used are hydralazine, which relaxes vascular smooth muscle, and prazosin which is an alpha-adrenergic blocking agent and dilates the resistance vessels in this way. Both of these agents cause a reflex tachycardia when given alone (hydralazine more than prazosin) but the use of beta-blocking agents has offset this and greatly increased the effectiveness of the vasodilators. These are potent drugs and the blood pressure of the vast majority of hypertensives is rendered acceptable by the triple combination therapy of diuretic, beta-blocker and vasodilator. It can be seen that with combination tablets plus a vasodilator the number of 'pills' that the patient has to take can be reduced to the minimum.

Hydralazine may cause a disseminated lupus erythematosus picture and the antinuclear factor should be checked before and during therapy. This seems to be dose dependent and is almost universal at 400 mg daily and above. Acetylator status should be determined as slow acetylators are more susceptible to the effects of the drug. The maximum dose should be restricted to about 200 mg per day.

Prazosin has a wider dose range and very large doses indeed are being used now (up to 40 mg per day). The initial dose may cause disastrous hypotension and the first tablet should be taken after going to bed. It causes less tachycardia than hydralazine. It is being superseded by newer, more predictable alpha-blocking drugs.

More recently the calcium antagonists such as verapamil and nifedipine have been advocated as vasodilators. As they seem to cause less reflex tachycardia their use has become more widespread especially in patients who are unsuitable for beta-blocking agents. Many physicians would now prefer nifedipine to other vasodilators such as hydralazine. Indeed combined beta-blocker/nifedipine tablets are available to improve compliance. Verapamil has many of the characteristics of a beta-blocker, e.g. slows heart rate and depresses myocardial contractility. When given intravenously together with a beta-blocker asystole can be produced. This has not been reported with oral preparations but since the drugs are so similar combined oral use is best avoided. A whole range of new calcium antagonists is becoming available and undoubtedly will increase the use of this group of agents. Minoxidil is a potent vasodilator and has a relatively long duration of action. It tends to cause hirsutism and for this reason is unsuitable for females. Like all the vasodilators it causes some fluid retention but this is possibly more marked with minoxidil. It is a drug that should probably only be used in refractory hypertension and by someone familiar with its use.

Centrally acting drugs

There are two centrally acting drugs in widespread use. These are methyldopa and clonidine. Both are rather old-fashioned drugs nowadays and methyldopa has been reported to have many side effects. In its time, however, it was the best available and many doctors, particularly those in general practice, still prescribe it. This is fully justified as methyldopa is a potent anti-hypertensive agent and many patients tolerate it well. The principal side effects are sedation and impotence but the former can be minimized by giving the drug in a single daily dose at night. The drug acts as a false transmitter at adrenergic nerve endings.

Clonidine also acts centrally. It may interfere with the baroreflex and has some central alpha-adrenergic blocking effects. It, too, can cause sedation but the principal problem is that if it is stopped abruptly the blood pressure may rebound to very high levels. Clonidine therapy should always be phased out with gradual reduction in the dose. It can be absorbed through the skin and patch preparations are available which may be useful in those who do not like taking tablets – quite a common problem in the management of hypertension.

Angiotensin converting enzyme (ACE) inhibitors

These are relatively new drugs which block conversion of angiotensin I to angiotensin II. They are also known, therefore, as converting enzyme inhibitors. This is not the sole mode of action and like the majority of anti-hypertensive agents just exactly how they work is not known. Initially they were reserved for the treatment of severe resistant or malignant hypertension but their use is becoming more widespread in less severely ill patients.

All ACE inhibitors can cause profound drops in blood pressure. This is especially likely to be true where the renin levels are high, e.g. in renal hypertension or in those already on diuretic therapy. Great care must be taken with their introduction. They are, however, extremely potent and well accepted. Many new ACE inhibitors are being introduced but those currently available include captoril, enalapril and lisinopril.

These drugs can be potentiated by adding in a diuretic. They also raise serum potassium levels so that when a thiazide diuretic is used potassium-sparing diuretics should not be used in addition. One major side effect is a dry irritating cough which all ACE inhibitors so far available can cause. ACE inhibitors are also used to treat heart failure (see chapter 10).

Other anti-hypertensive agents

Labetalol is a combined alpha- and beta-adrenoceptor blocking agent. It is an effective drug and used quite widely.

Reserpine depletes noradrenaline stores. It became notorious for causing depression but this effect was probably overstated.

Ganglion-blocking agents are no longer used but the post-ganglionic blocking drugs guanethidine, bethanidine and dibrisoquine still have a place in the management of severe hypertension. They all tend to cause postural hypotension.

● **Malignant hypertension**

In some patients hypertension runs an accelerated and worsening course. It may occur in long-standing hypertensives or develop over a relatively short period. If this latter is the case then a secondary cause such as phaeochromocytoma or renal artery stenosis should be sought. Malignant hypertension is characterized by very high blood pressures (diastolic greater than 130 mmHg) and by proteinuria. There is fibrinoid necrosis of the small arterioles and the optic fundi often show haemorrhages, exudates and papilloedema.

Clinical presentation

Malignant hypertension may be detected during routine blood pressure checks but because of the level of the pressure these patients are often symptomatic. This is a medical emergency and such patients should be admitted to hospital.

They may have noticed headaches (especially in the mornings) and visual upsets due to the changes in the optic fundi. They are often generally unwell with diminished appetite and loss of weight. Occasionally they present with a so-called hypertensive crisis. This can be either acute left ventricular failure or hypertensive encephalopathy. The failure is due to the heart being unable to cope with the very high pressure and peripheral resistance while encephalopathy is due to raised intracranial pressure, in itself secondary to the effects of fibrinoid necrosis in the blood vessels of the brain. Essentially the same thing is happening to the intracranial blood vessels as is being seen in the optic fundi.

In pregnancy eclampsia also represents a hypertensive crisis and presents both mother and fetus with very great risk.

Treatment of malignant hypertension

The essential element is to reduce the blood pressure. This need not be done precipitously and indeed strokes and other neurological damage have resulted from too precipitous drops in pressure in these patients. The target initially should be a diastolic pressure of 100–110 mmHg and a systolic pressure of less than 200 mmHg. This can be readily achieved by oral drugs such as atenolol or nifedipine. Seldom is parenteral treatment necessary. Later, over several days to weeks the blood pressure can be titrated down to more normal levels.

● **Treatment of hypertensive emergencies**

Again the aim is to lower the blood pressure and any lowering whatsoever will improve the situation. Here, however, time is of the essence and parenteral therapy may be used. Among the drugs that have been employed are diazoxide (now never given as a bolus) as an intravenous infusion, phentolamine, nitroprusside and labetalol. This latter is also a beta-blocking agent and so care is required in its use in heart failure. Careful monitoring of the blood pressure response is required in an intensive care unit and once again too precipitous reductions in pressure can themselves be dangerous. As soon as is convenient these patients are switched to oral therapy.

12

Other cardiovascular disorders

● **Infective endocarditis**

Infective endocarditis is the term now used to include subacute bacterial endocarditis (SBE) and acute bacterial endocarditis (ABE). SBE tends to develop in a previously abnormal heart while ABE may occur in patients with no previous cardiac abnormality.

Subacute bacterial endocarditis

This is a notoriously difficult condition to diagnose as the early symptoms are of vague ill health such as lack of appetite, loss of energy, nausea and weight loss. Diagnosis is usually delayed for this reason. Once suspected there are usually some helpful physical signs and these should be sought. The patient is usually anaemic, the fingers clubbed and splinter haemorrhages may be seen in the nailbeds of hands and toes. Painful nodules on the fingers also occur (Osler's nodes). The spleen may be moderately enlarged and there may be subconjunctival haemorrhages. Roth's spots, which are probably arteritic, may be seen in the fundi. Haematuria is present in about 60 per cent of patients and auscultation of the heart will reveal a murmur in about 85 per cent (*Fig.* 12.1).

It is posssible to have no cardiac murmurs yet have infective endocarditis. Depending on the degree of damage caused the patient may be in heart failure. This may change dramatically as valves perforate or chordae are destroyed. When healing takes place valves may scar and become more incompetent so it is important to watch these patients closely for some considerable time after their endocarditis is cured.

Certain conditions predispose to the development of SBE. It develops more readily when there is a jet of blood passing from a high pressure chamber to a low pressure chamber such as occurs with a ventricular septal defect or with mitral or aortic incompetence. SBE, therefore, is less common with such lesions as atrial septal defect or mitral stenosis. There must also be a bacteraemia such as that which occurs with dental extractions or fillings but often there is no definite history as to where the bacteraemia may have originated from.

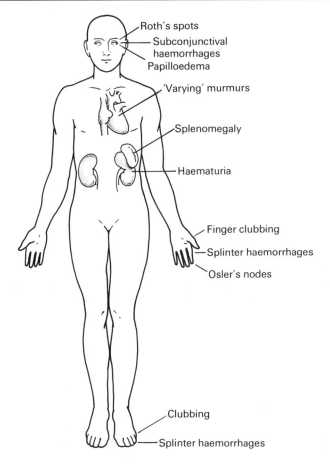

Fig. 12.1.   Features of subacute bacterial endocarditis.

Investigations

Echocardiography is helpful in up to 50 per cent of cases. Vegetations may be seen on the cusps of the mitral and aortic valves. Absence of echoes of vegetations cannot be taken as evidence against infective endocarditis.

Apart from the clinical findings the organism can usually be isolated from the blood stream (90 per cent). A maximum of six blood cultures should be taken over 24–48 hours before starting treatment. Further blood cultures do not increase the chances of identifying the organism. The ESR (or plasma viscosity) is raised, there is a normocytic normochromic anaemia and the white cell count is elevated. There is a concomitant immune reaction so that raised circulatory immune complexes are found while complement levels are reduced. Immune complexes settle out in the kidney and are the probable explanation of the haematuria so commonly present in these patients.

Infecting organisms

The spectrum of infecting organisms has changed over the years and now only about one-third of cases are due to *Streptococcus viridans* while the others largely comprise *Streptococcus epidermidis*, *Staphylococcus aureus* and *Streptococcus faecalis*.

Rarely the organisms are not grown from the blood stream. The usual cause of this is recent antibiotic therapy but occasionally it is due to odd infections such as Q-fever, chlamydia, fungi or anaerobes and the advice of the microbiologist should be sought in trying to identify them.

Prosthetic valves are rather prone to infective endocarditis and the organism can be introduced at the time of surgery. *Streptococcus epidermidis* and fungi are common culprits here.

Treatment

Depite modern antibiotics this is still a very serious condition. Mortality rates are still anything up to 30 per cent. After blood cultures are taken treatment is started with an aminoglycoside and large doses of penicillin intravenously. Subsequent antibiotic therapy can be tailored to the sensitivity of the organism. Cidal levels of the patient's plasma should be determined (i.e. a dilution of the patient's plasma of 1:8 or more should be capable of destroying the organism in culture). Treatment continues for at least 4 weeks (purely arbitrary – some would say shorter, some longer) and probably longer for patients with prosthetic valves. It is then our policy to allow the patients home after a few days, apyrexial off treatment, together with a temperature chart for them to record their own temperature over the next month. Any pyrexia and they return to be reassessed.

Some patients need emergency surgery to replace infected valves and this should be done sooner rather than later. Severe heart failure greatly increases the risks of surgery. Changing heart murmurs are described as characteristic of SBE and may indicate changes in the haemodynamic situation but in practice changing murmurs are relatively uncommon.

Acute bacterial endocarditis (ABE)

This is a much rarer condition and is more fulminant and severe. Many of the more chronic changes seen in SBE have not had time to develop so that anaemia is not so apparent, neither is haematuria nor splenomegaly. ABE usually develops on normal valves and is associated with overwhelming infection such as occurs in drug addicts, immunosuppressed individuals and it is also seen in children under the age of 2 years. *Staphylococcus aureus* is the common organism involved and there is a high overall mortality rate.

Marantic endocarditis

Marantic endocarditis is a form of endocarditis that develops in patients severely ill, usually with terminal cancer. It is usually largely overshadowed by the primary illness although in patients admitted *in extremis* acute bacterial endocarditis may be suspected especially if the echocardiogram shows vegetations on the valve cusps.

● **Cardiomyopathy**

When the heart muscle is diseased primarily, the condition is called a cardiomyopathy. There are three different types of cardiomyopathy: dilated, hypertrophic and restrictive.

Dilated cardiomyopathy

It is possible that some of these patients have previously had myocarditis, hypertension or have been alcoholic or perhaps even a combination of these. However, there are many patients where no such relationship could have occurred. Thyrotoxicosis is a rare cause.

One or other or both ventricles may be affected. It is by no means unusual for one ventricle, e.g. the left to be much more affected than the other. The clinical signs are those of failure of the relevant ventricle or of both ventricles. Bizarre rhythms and conduction defects are common on the ECG and sudden death often occurs. Treatment is as in right or left heart failure. Surprisingly in view of the failure beta-blockers have been used in treatment with some success. These must only be used under close supervision in hospital, at least initially, because while some patients improve on these drugs others worsen rapidly. Cautiously combined with vasodilators they may be more safe. Arrhythmias are treated as they arise and because the heart is dilated and akinetic anticoagulants are usually prescribed to try and minimize emboli and venous thrombosis. Some patients go on to cardiac transplantation if they are otherwise fit. Alcohol consumption should be kept to a minimum and if the cardiomyopathy is alcohol-induced there can be considerable improvement with abstinence. In the rare case due to thyrotoxicosis there can be dramatic improvement with appropriate treatment.

The prognosis is extremely variable and some patients may even get better. The vast majority, however, steadily deteriorate and die within a few years of diagnosis.

Hypertrophic cardiomyopathy

The characteristic pathology here is a thickened left ventricle such that the lumen becomes progressively obliterated (*Fig.* 12.2). The septum in particular is thick and relatively immobile. The right ventricle is sometimes affected and occasionally the pathology affects the right ventricle more than the left. The ventricle may clamp down on itself to such an extent that pressure gradients develop within different parts of it. Because of these obstructions of left ventricular outflow the condition is sometimes known as hypertrophic

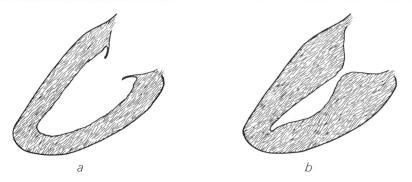

Fig. 12.2.   (a) Normal left ventricle. (b) Left ventricle in HOCM.

obstructive cardiomyopathy (HOCM), but in only 50 per cent of cases are left ventricular gradients present. It tends to run in families with an autosomal dominant pattern. These patients present with rhythm disturbances, angina, syncope, dyspnoea or are often detected by accident in the course of a routine chest X-ray or ECG. Left ventricular end diastolic pressure is increased because of the non-compliant muscle. The echocardiogram is the most helpful diagnostic aid (*Fig.* 12.3).

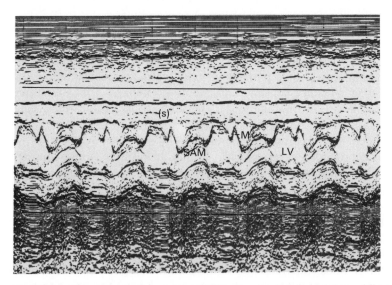

Fig. 12.3.   The echocardiogram in HOCM showing thickened, immobile septum (s), small left ventricular cavity (LV) and systolic anterior motion (SAM) of the mitral valve (M).

Treatment is with beta-blocking drugs. It is probably better not to use diuretics as an increased circulating blood volume is probably an advantage in this condition. Twenty-four-hour ECG tapes have shown these patients frequently to have had dangerous arrhythmias many of which are clinically not apparent. In view of this and the fact that sudden death is relatively common some cardiologists would use a drug such as amiodarone to lessen such abnormal rhythms, but the benefits of this therapy have yet to be established definitely..

Where obstruction and cavity obliteration are major features attempts have been made to remove some of the hypertrophied muscle surgically but the results have been disappointing. However, some patients with HOCM also have mitral reflux, and mitral valve replacement in some of them has had a beneficial effect. The major problem is now regarded as one of cardiac filling, i.e. blood returning to the heart is obstructed due to the stiff non-compliant ventricle. As a result heart failure finally ensues and treatment then becomes a compromise between that of hypertrophic cardiomyopathy (beta-blockers/verapamil) and heart failure (diuretics/vasodilators).

Restrictive cardiomyopathy

As the name suggests in this form of heart muscle disease there is restriction of cardiac filling. The clinical picture is very similar to constrictive pericarditis and even at cardiac catheterization it can be very difficult to separate these two conditions. It is much less common than the other two types of cardiomyopathy and amyloidosis is the commonest cause.

● **Aortic dissection**

This occurs when blood passes into the media of the aorta, destroys it and causes the intima and adventitia to separate. The process may be better thought of as a dissecting haematoma – a term that is gaining acceptance, and the general outcome is decided by where the haematoma finally extends and whether or not the aorta ruptures.

Most cases occur in previously hypertensive individuals but there are other associations with Marfan's syndrome, coarctation of the aorta, bicuspid aortic valve and, strangely, they may occur in the third trimester of pregnancy.

Three types have been described

Type I.   Affects the ascending aorta and around the arch (*Fig.* 12.4).

Type II.   Affects only the ascending aorta (*Fig.* 12.5).

Type III.   Affects the descending aorta (*Fig.* 12.6).

Not included in this classification are abdominal aortic aneurysms.

Of more practical importance is the knowledge as to whether the ascending or descending aorta is involved as the treatment differs between these two types.

The initial symptom is a tearing severe chest pain that resembles that of a myocardial infarction at least in part, but the ECG is normal. Pain in the

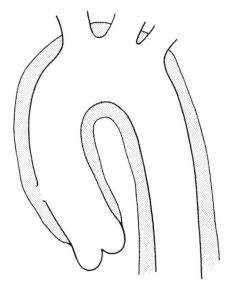

Fig. 12.4. Type I aortic dissection.

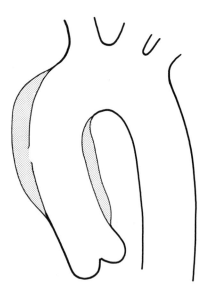

Fig. 12.5. Type II aortic dissection.

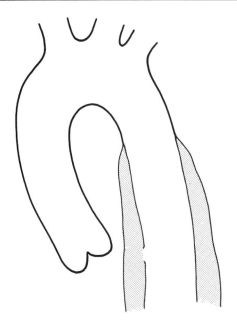

Fig. 12.6.   Type III aortic dissection.

anterior chest suggests the ascending aorta is involved while pain between the shoulder blades is more probably due to descending aortic involvement.

The dissecting haematoma may involve arteries, e.g. carotid, spinal, coronary and renal, as it goes on its way. It may cause the aortic valve to become incompetent and it may rupture into the pericardium or into the pleural space. Often it ruptures back into the aorta at some other point. The clinical signs depend on the pathology but, in all cases suggestive of dissection, bruits in the various arteries, e.g. carotid, should be sought and the early diastolic murmur of aortic incompetence listened for.

Investigations

The chest radiograph shows widening of the mediastinum or even a bulge on the aorta. The echocardiogram may show a double lumen and sometimes a flap can be identified within the aorta. Especially useful are computed tomographic (CT) and nuclear magnetic resonance (NMR) scans. It is seldom necessary to perform aortograms and these are not done without risk. The non-invasive scans should give all the information required.

The immediate management is absolute bed-rest, pain relief and prompt lowering of the blood pressure. Early surgical repair is advised in ascending aortic lesions. If a descending dissection involves vessels such as the renal or mesenteric arteries then sugical repair is indicated but otherwise these cases can be managed medically. In all cases whether managed medically or surgically the long-term control of the blood pressure is very important. It should be maintained at the lower end of the normal range.

● **Cardiac tumours**
Primary tumours of the heart are rare. They include lipomas, fibromas and rhabdomyomas but perhaps the commonest known is the myxoma. Malignant tumours also occur very rarely and include sarcomas and mesotheliomas. Secondary deposits are, however, common in the heart and are seen in up to 10 per cent of cancer victims at post mortem. Despite extensive invasion of the myocardium the clinical manifestations of cardiac involvement are often minimal.

Myxomas
These are almost always referred to as left atrial myxomas but they do occur in the right atrium as well and up to 5 per cent occur in the ventricles. They are difficult to detect clinically but there are usually general symptoms such as fatigue and tiredness, the ESR is raised and more specific manifestations such as arrhythmias, emboli or obstruction to blood flow through the heart may be presenting features. Often there are variable heart murmurs which may be altered by changes in posture. They are classically described as mimicking mitral stenosis although, of course, they have to be left atrial myxomas to do this. The echocardiogram is most useful and in left atrial myxomas coarse echoes will be seen under the mitral valve and in the left atrium. Two-dimensional echocardiography can often demonstrate the tumour flopping backwards and forwards. They are removed at surgery and there is a small recurrence rate.

● **Myocarditis**
Acute infections of the myocardium may be commoner than we thought. ECG abnormalities are often seen in patients with an acute infection and both the patient and his ECG fully recover. Where the infection leads to heart failure and rhythm or conduction disorders, these cases are much rarer.

Coxsackie B virus is the most important infecting agent in North America and Europe. At best it is uncommon. The patients may have chest pain and even ECG changes typical of a myocardial infarction. Pleuritic chest pain may also occur and heart failure may develop as may a variety of arrhythmias and conduction defects including ventricular tachycardia and fibrillation. Treatment is largely symptomatic.

Most recover completely although a small percentage go on to develop a picture indistinguishable from a dilated cardiomyopathy. It seems that exercise in increasing cardiac work may increase the damage to the heart so bed-rest in the acute phase and restriction of physical activities for some months thereafter is probably advisable.

In South America, Chagas' disease, due to *Trypanosoma cruzi*, produces an infective myocarditis, often in epidemic proportions. It may lead later on to a dilated cardiomyopathy and severe arrhythmias are common.

● Acute pericarditis

The clinical picture results from acute inflammation of the pericardium. Pain often develops which is retrosternal, tends to be sharp and may be partly pleuritic in character, worsening with respiration, and which, characteristically, is less severe when sitting up but worse when lying down.

A wide variety of conditions can cause pericarditis but viral infection, myocardial infarction and uraemia are probably the commonest. Pericarditis is seen to a varying extent with the rheumatic diseases, and several drugs can cause it as an adverse response, e.g. procainamide, quinidine and hydralazine.

On examination the characteristic pericardial rub is heard. This is very superficial and sounds nearer the stethoscope than do murmurs or heart sounds. It is scratchy in character and occurs in time with myocardial contraction. It often has a respiratory variation also as the heart moves with breathing and frequently there is some pleuritic involvement as well. The ECG is characteristic and shows ST segment elevation which is concave upwards. It is usually seen extensively throughout the unipolar and bipolar leads.

The prognosis is generally good and treatment is largely symptomatic, e.g. aspirin or indomethacin although, of course, the eventual outcome is largely determined by the initial cause. In viral pericarditis the ECG reverts to normal and it is doubtful if there are any long-term sequelae.

Pericardial effusion

Because the pericardium is a closed sac it is possible for fluid to gather within it. This often follows an inflammation of the pericardium but also occurs in heart failure or conditions, such as ruptured ventricle, where blood is allowed into the pericardial space. This sometimes occurs at cardiac catheterization and, probably commoner nowadays, at the time of insertion of temporary or permanent pacing electrodes.

Initially the pericardium will stretch but a point is reached where this can no longer occur and the heart then becomes compressed resulting in pericardial tamponade.

The clinical signs are those expected from a heart that cannot fill. The jugular venous pressure is elevated and tends to rise further with inspiration but this is more common with constrictive pericarditis. Similarly hepatomegaly, ascites and peripheral oedema develop only if the tamponade is chronic and are more commonly seen with constrictive pericarditis.

Pulsus paradoxus occurs. The usual inspiratory fall in blood pressure is more pronounced than normal and usually, on breathing, exceeds 10 mmHg. Note that this is not in fact paradoxical but just an amplification of what occurs in healthy people. The heart sounds are soft and distant and if the effusion results from pericarditis the pericardial rub, surprisingly, is still often heard.

On chest radiography the heart is large and globular, losing its normal anatomy and becoming much rounder. The ECG is low voltage and at cardiac catheterization a characteristic plateau is seen in diastolic ventricular pressure that reflects the impaired filling of the ventricle.

Echocardiography has proved most useful in detailing pericardial effusions. An echo-free space is seen behind the heart. It is also present anteriorly but is less easy to detect.

Many pericardial effusions will recover spontaneously, many are part of a terminal illness and due to secondary neoplasms but occasionally tamponade is severe enough to require drainage. Rarely, pericardial effusions are 'tapped' for diagnostic reasons.

Constrictive pericarditis

In constrictive pericarditis the pericardium is thick, stiff and in many cases may even be calcified. The heart is thus held in a rigid box-like structure and here, also, the clinical signs are those of impaired cardiac filling. Because the condition is much more chronic the physical signs such as ascites and hepatomegaly are often much more florid.

The jugular venous pressure increases moderately with inspiration (Kussmaul's sign). Despite the florid clinical signs the heart may be impalpable which would be very unusual if right heart failure were the cause of the ascites and oedema. A loud third heart sound (the pericardial knock) may be audible.

The ECG is low voltage, the echocardiograph may show dense echoes and the heart be shown to be relatively immobile. The heart is round on the chest radiograph but tends to be much smaller than in tamponade. A large round heart shadow, however, does not exclude constrictive pericarditis. Calcification may be seen in the pericardium and often shows up better on a lateral X-ray film. At catheterization the diastolic pressures are equal in all four chambers and there is the characteristic plateau pressure in the ventricles.

Classically constrictive pericarditis used to be a long-term sequela to acute tuberculous pericarditis. This is much less common now and most cases are of undetermined origin but trauma, rheumatoid arthritis, uraemia and neoplastic disease all occur.

Index